# Ethno-psychopharmacology

Advances in Current Practice

# Ethno-psychopharmacology

## Advances in Current Practice

Edited by

Chee H. Ng

Keh-Ming Lin

Bruce S. Singh

Edmond Y. K. Chiu

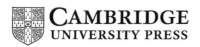

CAMBRIDGE UNIVERSITY PRESS
Cambridge, New York, Melbourne, Madrid, Cape Town, Singapore, São Paulo, Delhi

Cambridge University Press
The Edinburgh Building, Cambridge CB2 8RU, UK

Published in the United States of America by Cambridge University Press, New York

www.cambridge.org
Information on this title: www.cambridge.org/9780521873635

First published 2008

Printed in the United Kingdom at the University Press, Cambridge

*A catalog record for this publication is available from the British Library*

ISBN 978-0-521-87363-5 hardback

Chee Hong Ng dedicates this book to
the memory of Kim Leong Ng for being a lifetime mentor.

# Contents

# Figures

# Tables

# Contributors

**Chia-Hui CHEN, M.D.**
Division of Mental Health and Substance Abuse Research National Health Research Institutes, Taiwan

**Chun-Yu CHEN, M.S.**
Division of Mental Health and Substance Abuse Research National Health Research Institutes, Taiwan

**Jur-Shan CHENG, Ph.D.**
Center for Health Policy Research and Development, National Health Research Institutes, Taiwan

**Edmond Y.K. CHIU, A.M., M.B., B.S., D.P.M.**
Department of Psychiatry, University of Melbourne, Academic Unit for Psychiatry of Old Age, St George's Hospital, Victoria, Australia

**Deborah L. FLORES, M.D.**
David Geffen School of Medicine, Dept. of Psychiatry, Harbor-UCLA Medical Center Torrance, CA, USA

**Sang-Woo HAHN**
Department of Psychiatry, College of Medicine, Soonchunhyang University, Seoul, Korea

**Rhee-Hun KANG**
Department of Psychiatry, College of Medicine, Korea University, Seoul, Korea

**Steven KLIMIDIS, Ph.D.**
Centre for International Mental Health, School of Population Health, The University of Melbourne, Victoria, Australia

**Timothy LAMBERT, B.Sc., M.B., B.S., Ph.D., F.R.A.N.Z.C.P.**
Department of Psychological Medicine, University of Sydney, Royal Prince Alfred Hospital, Camperdown NSW, Australia

**William B. LAWSON, M.D., Ph.D., F.A.P.A.**
Department of Psychiatry, Howard University Hospital, Washington, DC, USA

**Min-Soo LEE, M.D., Ph.D.**
Department of Psychiatry, Korea University College of Medicine, Seoul, Korea

**Keh-Ming LIN, M.D., M.P.H.**
Division of Mental Health and Substance Abuse Research, National Health Research Institutes, Taiwan

**Mario MAJ, M.D.**
Department of Psychiatry, University of Naples, Naples, Italy

**Ricardo MENDOZA, M.D.**
David Geffen School of Medicine at UCLA,
Department of Psychiatry, Harbor-UCLA
Medical Center, Torrance, CA, USA

**Juan E. MEZZICH, M.D., Ph.D.**
International Center for Mental Health and
Division of Psychiatric Epidemiology, Mount
Sinai School of Medicine, New York
University, New York, USA

**Chee H. NG, M.B., B.S., M.Med., M.D.**
Department of Psychiatry, The University of
Melbourne, St Vincent Hospital & The
Melbourne Clinic, Victoria, Australia

**Trevor R. NORMAN, B.Sc., Ph.D.**
Department of Psychiatry, University of
Melbourne, Austin Hospital, Victoria,
Australia

**M. Angeles RUIPEREZ, Ph.D.**
Department of Psychobiology and Basic and
Clinical Psychology, Universitat Jaume I.
Castelló, Spain

**Norman SARTORIUS, M.D., Ph.D.**
Geneva, Switzerland

**Isaac SCHWEITZER, M.B., B.S., D.P.M.,
F.R.A.N.Z.C.P., M.D.**
Department of Psychiatry, The University of
Melbourne, Professorial Unit, The
Melbourne Clinic, Victoria, Australia

**Tian-Mei SI, M.D., Ph.D.**
Institute of Mental Health, Peking University
Beijing, China

**Bruce S. SINGH, M.B., B.S., Ph.D.**
Department of Psychiatry, University of
Melbourne, Royal Melbourne Hospital,
Victoria, Australia

**Chay-Hoon TAN, M.B., B.S., M.Med., Ph.D.**
Department of Pharmacology, National
University of Singapore, Kent Ridge,
Singapore

**Pichet UDOMRATN, M.D.**
Department of Psychiatry, Faculty of
Medicine, Prince of Songkla University, Hat
Yai, Songkhla, Thailand

**Helena VILLA, Ph.D.**
Department of Psychobiology and Basic and
Clinical Psychology, Universitat Jaume I.
Castelló, Spain

**Sheng-Chang WANG, M.D., M.Sc.**
Division of Mental Health and Substance
Abuse Research National Health Research
Institutes, Taiwan

**Shu-Han YU, M.D.**
Division of Mental Health and Substance
Abuse Research National Health Research
Institutes, Taiwan

**Xin YU, M.D.**
Institute of Mental Health, Peking University
Beijing, China

# Foreword

This book is very important for two reasons: it is the first-ever textbook of psychopharmacology focusing on the Asia-Pacific region, and it is, as far as I know, the first internationally authored volume dealing specifically with ethno-psychopharmacology.

Both developments are remarkable. In the past few years, the international literature has been enriched by textbooks of psychiatry focusing on Latin America, Asia and Africa, which have proved to be very useful to clinicians in the respective regions, while at the same time providing the international readership with a lot of previously unavailable information. If these textbooks have been useful, even more timely may be this first "regional" textbook of psychopharmacology, which is likely to improve psychiatric practice in the Asia-Pacific region and represent a model for other regions of the world.

On the other hand, a book on ethno-psychopharmacology, which could perhaps have been regarded as a scientific curiosity a decade ago, will certainly not be perceived as such today by the vast majority of psychiatrists worldwide. Most of us live now in multiethnic environments, in which cultural variations in the expression of psychopathology can be directly observed by the average practitioner, and in which problems in communication and diagnostic approach to persons with different ethnic and cultural backgrounds are being experienced on a daily basis. Increasingly widespread also is the awareness of the ethnic and cultural variations in the response to the most common psychotropic medications, which is certainly a matter of genetic polymorphisms, but also a consequence of the impact of a variety of environmental factors.

Nowadays most trials of psychotropic drugs are multicentric, and an increasing number of them are carried out in different regions of the world. However, ethnic variations in response to the tested drugs are rarely a focus of attention in these trials. Moreover, treatment guidelines produced in North America and Europe are often regarded as universally valid, and rarely adapted to other regional contexts. This is still partly due to some reluctance to accept the concept of ethnic variability, as if it were "politically incorrect." I have a vivid recollection of what happened not many years ago at an international psychiatric meeting, in which a prominent expert who had briefly mentioned in his presentation the issue of ethnic variation in drug response was subtly accused in the subsequent discussion to be racist. What should be regarded as racist today, instead, is trying to transfer automatically the information acquired in specific areas of the world to all other cultures and ethnicities, even if this implies the use of doses of medications that are inappropriate or of treatment schedules that are not transferable.

This book is a real treasure of information and ideas for research in the field of ethno-psychopharmacology. I think it should be welcomed by clinicians and by researchers in psychiatry and psychopharmacology in all regions of the world. It is unique in the current scientific literature, and is likely to remain as such for many years.

Mario Maj
President Elect, World Psychiatric Association

# Acknowledgments

The editors wish to acknowledge the following persons: Christine Hua-Chun Chang and Amy Chia-Hui Lin, secretaries to Keh-Ming Lin; Fiona Kelly, personal assistant to Bruce Singh; and Joy Preston, personal assistant to Edmond Chiu.

# Introduction

Isaac Schweitzer

It has often been claimed that modern psychopharmacology began with the discovery of chlorpromazine in 1952. Australian psychiatrists argue that the legitimate date is 1949 with the landmark publication by John Cade detailing a case series of ten manic patients who had responded dramatically to lithium salts. The veracity of this argument is supported by the fact that lithium remains the gold standard for bipolar disorder treatment whereas chlorpromazine use for schizophrenia is rapidly disappearing. The genius of John Cade has recently been further highlighted by conversations I have had with one of the editor's of this volume, Edmond Y. K. Chiu, who was my clinical supervisor during 1977. I was a young psychiatric registrar working in an academic unit in Melbourne, Australia. I have clear recollections of Chiu enlightening me that Asian patients were more vulnerable to experiencing side effects to lithium and tricyclic antidepressants and would often respond well to lower doses than the average Caucasian. Chiu, who was born in Hong Kong, informs me that he learned this from Cade. It was in 1968 when as a trainee psychiatrist he came to work with Cade in Melbourne. On his return to Hong Kong, his treatment of his Chinese patients benefited by improved compliance and response rates, having followed Cade's astute observations of the ethnic differences in drug handling of psychotropics.

Should we therefore credit the birth of the discipline of ethno-psychopharmacology to Cade? There is little doubt that since the introduction of modern-day psychotropic medications, there have been many astute clinicians from around the world who have made similar observations regarding ethnic differences in response and tolerability of psychiatric treatments. We must therefore ask, why if this issue has been recognized for such a long time, has there been relatively little research in this area. Few pharmaceutical companies have embarked on such investigations for their products. Most governmental regulatory requirements do not specify a need

*Ethno-psychopharmacology: Advances in Current Practice*, eds. C. H. Ng, K.-M. Lin, B. S. Singh and E. Y. K. Chiu. Published by Cambridge University Press. © C. H. Ng, K.-M. Lin, B. S. Singh and E. Y. K. Chiu 2008.

for such research prior to approving new medications for release. Have we remained ethnocentric in our perspectives – what is good for one is good for all? Does the answer lie in our sensitivity to the dictum that "all men are created equal" and in acknowledging ethnic differences in responses to medication we are somehow challenging this dictum?

The word "ethnicity" is closely aligned with "race" and when racial differences are discussed, associations with white supremacist movements and the like are made; this evokes strong emotional reactions in most of us. The linking of fields such as eugenics and Nazi Germany's extermination program has resulted in this area being largely discarded by the scientific community. These issues are a potential minefield and may have acted as significant barriers to embarking on this area of endeavour. But the fact the science has been abused to justify political persecution in the past should not be a barrier to exploring the field as new findings emerge.

As human beings we share many similarities, we are much more alike than are our differences; over 99% of our genes are the same in all human beings. At the same time we do vary, individually and according to our social groupings. When we live in groups, particularly over many generations, our genes come to be more closely aligned, more likely to share certain similarities and develop differences to other social groups. In addition, our lifestyle, diet and other customs are more closely related. It is such concepts of ethnicity that encompass the essence of ethno-psychopharmacology, as espoused by Keh-Ming Lin, the pioneer and leading proponent of the field and one of the editors of this volume.

Ethno-psychopharmacology is attempting to answer the questions of how culture and genetic differences of natural social groupings of the human race determine and influence response to psychotropic medications. The prefix "ethno" has been chosen as it encompasses both the genetic and cultural differences of social groupings, the concept of race becoming increasingly an obsolete one.

It is interesting to note that despite cultural differences the stigma associated with psychiatric disorder has been universally observed. One form this has taken is the trivialization and minimization of psychiatric conditions; they are frequently dismissed as being mild, unimportant and not serious enough to be worthy of treatment. Several worldwide studies have shown psychiatric disorders to be not only highly prevalent but also amongst the most disabling of illnesses, impacting severely on loss of productivity and reducing quality of life. The Global Burden of Disease Study commissioned by the World Health Organization (WHO) predicts that by 2020, depression will have become the second largest contributor of disease burden worldwide. However, we have made many wonderful psychopharmacological discoveries over the past 60 years. We are now beginning to address those critical issues of how best to make these life-saving discoveries available to all populations. If medicine is to be successful in this endeavour a very thorough understanding of the influence of culture and genetic variation on societies throughout the world is required.

In this volume, the reader will have access to a practical guide to the current advances in ethno-psychopharmacology with a particular focus on the Asia-Pacific region. Genetic factors that control both pharmacokinetics and pharmacodynamics of psychotropic drugs are subject to marked variation between individuals and ethnic groups. These clinically significant issues are related to genetic polymorphisms in drug metabolism particularly affecting CYP2D6 and CYP2C19. For instance, about 15–30% of Asians are poor metabolizers of CYP2C19 compared to 3–6% of Caucasians and 2–4% of Africans. The deficient genotypes are prevalent in Asian populations. In the case of CYP2D6, about 5–10% of Caucasians are poor metabolizers in contrast to only 1–2% of Asians. However, up to 50% of Asians carry a mutant allele that is an intermediate functioning allele. This gives rise to a high incidence of intermediate metabolizers with reduced metabolic capacity. Pharmacodynamic factors are similarly found to have a significant role in drug response but these have been less studied. Candidate genes related to pharmacodynamic effects include those coding for receptors (dopamine, noradrenaline and serotonin receptors) and drug transporters (serotonin).

Response to pharmacotherapy is multifaceted and involves the interaction of genetic, environmental and cultural factors. Environmental factors play a clinically significant role in determining the pharmacokinetics of psychotropic medications but are often inadequately considered. A range of environmental factors, including dietary factors, herbal medication, concomitant medication and other substances, significantly modifies the expression of the genes influencing pharmacokinetics and pharmacodynamics. Dietary factors, herbal medication, chemicals and pollutants are exogenous agents that may alter the activity of drug metabolizing enzymes particularly CYP2D6, CYP1A2 and CYP3A4. Sociocultural considerations represent a diverse dimension affecting pharmacotherapeutic response. Cross-cultural issues can affect diagnosis, beliefs and expectations concerning treatment, compliance, and placebo effect and can impact upon drug response in ways that may be more potent than biological mechanisms. Furthermore, prescribing patterns of the clinician may often determine the type and the dosage of the medication during treatment initiation and maintenance, which may lead to differences in response.

This volume covers topics including cultural perspectives in psychiatric diagnosis and psychopharmacotherapy, differences in pharmacokinetics and pharmacodynamics of psychotropics, pharmacogenetics of ethnic populations, ethnic variations in psychotropic responses, complementary medicines in mental disorders, attitudes towards psychotropic medications, prescribing practices in Asia-Pacific countries, pharmaco-economic implications, integrating theory and practice, and future research directions. The aim of this volume is to update the clinicians with important research findings that will influence their clinical practice, as well as providing researchers with a comprehensive overview of contemporary research directions and where the field is heading. This volume challenges clinicians, pharmacologists, geneticists and social anthropologists to continue their explorations in this field and to increase our understanding of the effects of ethnicity on psychopharmacological science and practice.

## 2

# Culture and psychopathology

Juan E. Mezzich, M. Angeles Ruiperez, and Helena Villa

## Introduction

The traditional Western conceptualization of mental disorders as individual experiences that have little or nothing to do with social, cultural or ethnic components, together with the pre-eminence attained in the study of the human brain over the last decades of the twentieth century, have resulted in an increase in the number of biological or intrapsychic explanations put forward by contemporary psychopathology. In consequence, how sociocultural processes are involved in explaining and understanding psychopathological manifestations is not very clearly defined (Agbayani-Siewert, Takeuchi & Pangan, 1999; Fábrega, 1995).

Nevertheless, parallel to this, there has also been a growing and renewed interest in understanding the role played by culture in mental disorders in order to allow cultural aspects to be included in the conceptualization of psychopathologies, in the light of the results obtained by a large number of research studies (for a review, see López & Guarnaccia, 2005).

This interest in seeking to achieve the integration and interaction of biopsychosocial variables within the explanation of psychopathological behavior represented the beginning of a change of paradigm as regards the explanation of both normal and psychopathological human behavior (Mezzich, Lewis-Fernández & Ruipérez, 2003). This change in paradigm involves accepting the fact that psychic phenomena can be explained on a molecular and cellular level, involving tissues, organs, systems, the organism, the way information is processed, the physical surroundings or the sociocultural context (Cacioppo & Berntson, 1992, 2006; Mezzich et al., 2003; Westen, 2004).

Failing to take the cultural perspective into account can therefore mean that normal variations in the behavior of persons belonging to one culture are seen

*Ethno-psychopharmacology: Advances in Current Practice*, eds. C. H. Ng, K.-M. Lin, B. S. Singh and E. Y. K. Chiu. Published by Cambridge University Press. © C. H. Ng, K.-M. Lin, B. S. Singh and E. Y. K. Chiu 2008.

as being pathological from another cultural perspective. This chapter attempts to provide empirical evidence concerning the weight that some of these cultural context-related variables have in the manifestation of mental disorders.

First, we are going to briefly review some of the terms used to refer to ethnic differences and to describe the processes that take place when two or more cultural groups come into contact with each other. Second, we will outline some studies that illustrate how cultural aspects can affect, for example, the prevalence of certain disorders, the different ways symptoms are manifested, how therapeutic aid is sought or the efficacy of different forms of treatment. Cultural aspects can determine the appearance of syndromes that are specific to each culture (culture-bound syndromes) or can affect the manifestation of the symptoms that make up the different mental disorders. We will then show how cultural variations have been incorporated into the different systems of classification. Last, we will also detail the current recommendations on including cultural aspects in the diagnoses of mental disorders.

## Some concepts used in transcultural research

Before going on to analyze the importance of taking cultural factors into account in order to correctly identify symptoms and, therefore, to reach a correct diagnosis and apply a suitable treatment, we are going to briefly review some of the terms frequently used to talk about cultural factors, such as race or ethnicity, as well as acculturation. Despite their widespread use both by laypersons and in academic spheres, these terms have rarely been defined and on occasions are even used indistinctly (Adebimpe, 1994).

### Culture

This is a term that is widely used with a number of different meanings, with no generally agreed definition having been formulated to date. For example, Allen (1992) made a distinction between seven different uses of the term "culture," i.e., generic, expressive, hierarchical, superorganic, holistic, pluralistic and hegemonic. The most pragmatic use of the term refers to culture as a set of guidelines or formulae that allow intercommunication with the surroundings (MacLachlan, 1997).

### Race

This term was initially considered as referring to an unalterable biological category, based on distinguishing groups according to shared genetic characteristics. Yet, the evidence for basing racial categorization on biological grounds is weak and frequently conflictive (Williams, Yu & Jackson, 1997) and biology-based racial classifications (although often thought to be valid and scientific) tend to vary arbitrarily depending on the social, political and economic climate, as well as on social and cultural prejudices.

## Ethnicity

This term is used to refer to a group of persons who share a geographical area, nationality or cultural inheritance (Berreman, 1991), and hence it has been suggested that, as humans, we are not born as members of a particular ethnic group but instead it may be a characteristic that has to be learned. This being the case, socializing oneself within a particular ethnic group will include learning aspects such as language, lifestyles, prejudices, daily activities, values, and so forth (Berreman, 1991).

Human migratory movements, which have led to the mixing of cultures, are another aspect to be taken into account from a cultural perspective. Although these migratory movements have facilitated the progress of humanity, from the individual and group point of view they entail a psychological and social impact that has aroused a great deal of scientific interest. It is therefore important to analyze the processes that take place when various groups of humans come into contact with each other.

Unfortunately, the empirical research that has been conducted in this area has been affected by differences in the methodological rigor and the diversity of theoretical postures employed. Two broad approaches stand out among the different theoretical standpoints: (a) the earlier theories, which posited that being an immigrant always involved marginalization phenomena, and (b) the more modern theories, which conceived immigration experiences in more positive and adaptive terms.

The studies conducted from this latter perspective seek to explain the psychological and social phenomena that are produced during the process in which an individual or group belonging to one ethnic group (generally the minority) must become part of another culture (generally the majority). Psychopathology focuses its attention on analyzing the relation between the process of immigration and the manifestation of psychopathological behaviors. In order to understand such a process two clearly distinct elements must be borne in mind – those that refer to the individual and/or group responses that are produced during the process (acculturation and adaptation) and those that allude to the characteristics of the cultures that come into contact.

## Acculturation

Findings from research into psychological acculturation have defined three levels, and claim that psychological changes can range from very easy to very complicated: *non-conflictive psychological acculturation* (when the demands in the process of acculturation are limited to learning new behavioral repertoires that are appropriate for the new cultural context), *cultural shock* or *acculturative stress* (when the individuals do not find it easy to change their behavioral repertoires and/or acquire new ones, and experience a certain amount of emotional malaise) and *psychopathological disorders* (when the changes in the cultural context exceed the individuals' capacities to cope, either due to their magnitude, the speed with which they come about or other features in the process, which trigger severe psychological problems such as clinical depression and anxiety).

## Adaptation

In the broad sense of the term, adaptation refers to the changes that take place in individuals or groups in response to the demands imposed by their surroundings. Recent literature has analyzed the distinction between psychological adaptation and sociocultural adaptation (Berry *et al.*, 2006; Sam *et al.*, 2006; Searle & Ward, 1990; Ward & Kennedy, 1999). Psychological adaptation, on the one hand, refers to the set of internal psychological responses, including a clear personal and cultural sense of identity, good mental health and personal satisfaction in the new cultural context. Sociocultural adaptation, on the other hand, refers to the set of external psychological responses that individuals give in their new cultural context, including skills they need so as to be able to cope with the problems that crop up in their daily activities, especially in the family, social and work areas.

Although empirical studies usually present and explain these two forms of adaptation using the same theoretical assumptions, there are reasons to believe that they are conceptually different. This distinction is made on the grounds that psychological adaptation can be analyzed better within a psychopathological approach whereas sociocultural adaptation would be better dealt with by the social skills theories (Ward, 1996).

## Relation between the two cultures

As a result of immigration, many societies become culturally plural. Yet, in most cases the groups do not have the same power (as regards numbers, economy or politics). All plural societies need to address the issue of how the acculturation process takes place, at both the cultural group level and at that of their members.

In order to understand the relations that are established between the dominant group and the non-dominant group, Berry (1997) claims that it is necessary to consider two issues at the same time. First, to what extent is it important to maintain one's cultural identity and its characteristics? And, second, to what extent must immigrants integrate into other cultural groups, thus losing their own original culture?

In addressing these two questions, Berry (1997) considers that four acculturation strategies are generated from the point of view of the non-dominant group, and these can be represented as the two poles of a continuum: *assimilation* (when the individuals do not want to maintain their cultural identity and seek daily inter-actions with the dominant culture), *separation* (when the individuals grant an excessively high value to their own culture and at the same time wish to avoid con-tact with the dominant culture), *integration* (when there is a desire to maintain the original culture and to develop interactions with the host culture) and *marginaliza-tion* (when there is little chance or interest to maintain their own culture and little desire to forge relationships with others). Berry's (1997) integration corresponds to the term *biculturality* used to refer to the situation in which individuals identify themselves simultaneously with two cultures that are in contact and are competent in both of them (Cameron & Lalonde, 1994; Szapocznil & Kurtines, 1993) and will only occur in societies that are explicitly multicultural.

At the present time there is no universally accepted research model and thus, in spite of the large number of studies carried out over the past 30 years, the lack of a single conceptual field that is common to all of them makes it difficult to compare their findings and in fact on many occasions the results from these studies even contradict one another.

Thus, some studies conducted to research into biculturalism and psychopathol-ogy show that an individual who lives between two cultures can undergo a number of different psychopathological alterations due to the continual need to adapt to each of them whenever the cultural demands require them to do so (Cheng, Lee & Benet-Martínez, 2006). Other studies, however, show that individuals who live in two cultures may experience greater benefits than if they were to live a mono-cultural lifestyle (Blackledge, 2003). Berry (2006), on the other hand, concludes that the key to enjoying psychological well-being lies in the ability to develop and maintain cultural competencies in both cultures.

In view of the different manifestations of psychopathological behaviors found in diverse groups that cannot be adequately accounted for by factors concerning race, ethnic group or the acculturation process, Agbayani-Siewert *et al.* (1999) put forward a model that allows direct examination of the impact of cultural factors on psychopathological manifestations, while continuing to include structural social factors.

In this line, Hofstede (1980) conducted a transcultural study in which five rele-vant psychological dimensions were identified empirically in all the cultures that were studied, i.e. power–distance (from small to large), collectivism–individualism, femininity–masculinity, uncertainty avoidance (from weak to strong) and time orientation (from short term to long term).

Thus, analyzing the individualism/collectivism construct as a cultural factor can help to explain why some ethnic groups apparently under-use mental health services and, in contrast, rely on members of the family to provide care in possible cases of mental illness. Individualism emphasizes autonomy and priority is given to personal goals over those of the group. Collectivists, however, do not generally see personal or individual problems as being important enough to seek professional help because they tend to rely on collective ways of coping as a means of making life changes easier to deal with (Triandis, 1993). Taking the collectivist/individualist construct into account therefore goes beyond racial or ethnic categories, and so it is better able to explain the cultural structures that affect perceptions, expressions and responses to the psychopathology.

## Influence of culture on the prevalence and expression of symptoms

Although some forms of psychopathological expression can be universal, cultural aspects can affect the manifestation of certain symptoms and, in consequence, the prevalence of a mental disorder (Alegria, Takeuchi, Canino *et al.*, 2004; Chang, 2002). Thus, at this point we are going to review briefly the studies that have attempted to explain the relation between cultural aspects and the expression of psychological malaise. In these studies it becomes clear that the lack of a single generally agreed theoretical model gives rise to dissimilar results because most of them use either ethnic or racial categories or categories related to acculturation processes (structural factors) to explain how culture shapes the perception and expression of the psychopathology, while offering little information about the role played by cultural factors (Agbayani-Siewert *et al.*, 1999).

One strategy that is commonly used to understand the impact of cultural factors on mental illnesses has been to describe the distribution of mental illnesses among different racial and ethnic categories. Because these early studies were carried out on the emigrant population in the USA in the late nineteenth and early twentieth century, a debate began as to whether the relation between particular ethnic groups and psychopathology was due to the stress caused by emigration itself, to a self-selection of persons who were susceptible to certain psychiatric disorders in emigrants or to factors that were specific to an ethnic group (Collazos *et al.*, 2005).

The consistency of the findings from this early research, as regards the higher prevalence of schizophrenia and lower rates of affective disorders among Afro-Americans, led to suggestions that there was little biological foundation for feelings of sadness and depression in Afro-Americans, in addition to a certain predisposition towards schizophrenia that could be attributed to race (Bevis, 1921). Yet, later reviews of these studies reveal the presence of errors in the methodologies used, such as the low degree of reliability of the diagnoses or failing to take into account other variables that could account for such differences (e.g. age, cultural level, socioeconomic level) (Bell & Mehta, 1980). In a similar way, the fact that

Afro-Americans were over-represented among the lower economic levels could mean that this susceptibility to mental disorders was due to stressors related to poverty and not to the presence of a vulnerability that could be attributed to ethnic or racial factors (Williams, 1986).

Another variable that was neglected in these early studies was the weight given to cultural factors in the use of mental health services. This is especially important in the case of Asian-Americans, who grant so much importance to support from the family that it is quite incompatible with western forms of treatment. As a result, the fact that this population makes little use of mental health services has been (wrongly) interpreted as being a sign of good psychological adjustment (Kimmich, 1960; Kitano, 1962; Sue & Kirk, 1975; Yamamoto, James & Palley, 1968).

From the above, it becomes clear that simplistic interpretations of the results of the studies into psychopathology and culture in the literature must be avoided, while at the same time efforts must also be made to develop a more refined methodology that involves a careful analysis of the factors that condition such a relationship (Collazos *et al.*, 2005).

As regards the expression of symptoms, several studies have suggested that the symptomatic expressions of specific disorders may vary depending on the patients' culture (Adebimpe, Chu & Klein, 1982). Marsella (1988) suggested that the biological bases of a disorder and the influence of the environment on the clinical picture were inversely proportional to each other. Thus, a disorder produced mainly by biological forces (such as a stroke) will have less intercultural variability than a disorder primarily due to social or environmental causes (such as a dissociative disorder). On the other hand, psychotic and mood disorders, which have important biological determining factors but are also strongly influenced by the sociocultural surroundings, should lie somewhere between the two extremes as regards their degree of transcultural variability.

The role played by culture in the expression of symptoms, as well as in the greater acceptance of certain forms of psychopathological expression, is especially well illustrated in the studies conducted on depression among the Hutterites, on neurasthenia in China and on nervous breakdowns in the Puerto Rican population.

### The Hutterites

The Hutterites are members of a Baptist sect originally from Central Europe, whose ancestors were forced to emigrate after being subjected to important religious persecutions in the sixteenth century. They have remained isolated in religious communes in both the United States and Canada and therefore constitute a homogenous social group that is especially interesting for separating cultural factors from structural factors.

In a study promoted by the National Institute of Mental Health (NIMH) the Hutterites showed high rates of psychosis (Eaton & Weil, 1955). Nevertheless, a later re-analysis of the data using DSM-III-R diagnostic criteria (American Psychiatric Association [APA], 1980) showed that the rate of major depression was four times higher than that of schizophrenia (Torrey, 1995).

These latter results, together with the observation by Eaton and Weil (1955) that the contents of the deliria were spiritual or religious and that all of them involved God, seemed to indicate that the lifestyle of the Hutterites favored the expression of psychological malaise as depression. The Hutterites believed that depression could only be experienced by "good folk," and therefore suffering this disorder was not seen as being a stigmatization. It seems, then, that the type of depression described in the Hutterites was a common reaction to their lifestyle and it has thus been taken as a classic example of the profound influences of culture on the way these individuals respond to the environment, as well as on the acceptance of such a response by the group.

## Neurasthenia in China

The main source of error in the interpretation of transcultural epidemiological studies stem from what Kleinman (1977) called category fallacy, which refers to the failure to identify certain symptoms as a consequence of using culturally irrelevant diagnostic instruments. This is what, according to Kleinman (1977), Lin (1982) and Zhang (1995), would account for the low rates of depressive disorders in the Chinese population compared to the high rates of neurasthenia found in some studies (Cheung, 1989; Ming-Yuan, 1989).

Somatic upsets are the primary symptoms of depression among the Chinese, in contrast to the affective and dysphoric manifestations that are more common in the West (Cheung & Bernard, 1982; Kleinman, 1977, 1988; Marsella, Kinzie & Gordon, 1973; Tseng, 1975).

On the other hand, the concept of neurasthenia, which was introduced by the American neurologist George Beard in 1869, characterized a syndrome that included physical symptoms and mental fatigue, loss of memory, insomnia, palpitations, dizziness, hypochondria, depressive moods, phobias and headaches, among others. This term, despite its popularity from the nineteenth century up to the mid twentieth century, stopped being used following the publication of the DSM-III in 1980, as this manual did not include the diagnosis of neurasthenia and its defining symptoms were spread out over other categories such as depression, anxiety and somatoform disorders. Despite the APA's decision to exclude neurasthenia from the DSM-III (and later editions), this category is still present in Chinese psychiatric nosology.

Kleinman (1986) claimed that neurasthenia was a cultural form of chronic somatization that outlined several different types of psychopathological disorders, the major depressive disorder included in western classifications being the one that best accounted for this disorder. This would explain the lower rate of prevalence of the diagnosis of "depressive disorder" among the Chinese population.

## Ataque de nervios

Another example of error in the estimation of the prevalence of certain disorders by using systems of diagnosis that fail to take cultural characteristics into account is the case of *ataque de nervios* among Puerto Ricans.

In a transcultural study conducted in the eighties it was found that Puerto Ricans displayed a greater number of somatic symptoms than other ethnic groups. Later, Guarnaccia, Angel, and Woobey (1989) reviewed the data from the epidemiologic catchment area (ECA) study by applying an instrument designed to consider the existence of *ataque de nervios* (a culture-dependent syndrome that expresses personal malaise in the Puerto Rican population and some other groups of Latinos). Findings showed that the "excessive" somatic symptoms observed when using the Diagnostic Interview Schedule (DIS) structured interview were related to the presence of *ataque de nervios* in this population – a syndrome the DIS interview does not contemplate and therefore could not detect (Guarnaccia *et al.*, 1989).

After reviewing these studies we can conclude that cultural aspects not only affect the expression of malaise, but also the fact that failing to take them into account can hinder the capacity to identify malaise in a subject from another culture (Guarnaccia *et al.*, 1989; Malgady, Rogler & Cortes, 1996). These categories of cultural malaise were defined by Rubel (1964) as "a coherent set of symptoms within a particular population, whose members display similar patterns of response" and since they were identified, different terms have been used to label them: idioms of distress, disorders specific to a particular culture, popular syndromes, syndromes that are "linked" or "reactive" to a culture, and ethnic or exotic psychoses, among others. This type of syndrome is currently grouped under the term *culture-bound syndromes.*

## Culture-bound syndromes

The unprecedented inclusion of culture-bound syndromes in the DSM-IV (APA, 1994) highlights the need to study such syndromes and the chance to develop a research plan that allows a careful, thorough study of the issue. The DSM-IV contains symptomatic descriptions of 25 culture-bound syndromes developed by the Culture and Diagnosis Group (Mezzich *et al.*, 1996), as well as including the definition of culture-bound syndrome.

The term culture-bound syndrome denotes recurrent, locality-specific patterns of aberrant behavior and troubling experience that may not be linked to a particular DSM-IV diagnostic category. Many of these patterns are indigenously considered to be "illnesses" or at least afflictions, and most have local names. Although presentations conforming to the major DSM-IV categories can be found throughout the world, the particular symptoms, course, and social response are very influenced by local cultural factors. In contrast, culture-bound syndromes are generally limited to specific societies or culture areas and are localized, folk, diagnostic categories that frame coherent meanings for certain repetitive, patterned, and troubling sets of experiences and observations. (Mezzich *et al.*, 1996, p. 844)

The culture-bound syndromes listed in DSM-IV (APA, 1994) are: *amok, ataque de nervios, bilis and colera, boufe delirante*, brain fag, *dhat*, falling out or blacking out, ghost sickness, *hwa-byung, koro, latah, locura, mal de ojo, nervios, pibloktoq, qigong psychotic reaction, rootwork, sangue dormido, shenjing shuairo* (neurasthenia), *shen-k'uei (shenkui), shin-byung*, spell, *susto, taijin kyofusho*, zar.

As stated in the Latin American Guide for Psychiatric Diagnosis (GLDP, from the Spanish name) (Latin American Psychiatric Association [APAL], 2004), there are other syndromes that little is known about because of the absence of epidemiological studies that focus on the reliability of their clinical descriptions. In this same vein, Guarnaccia and Rogler (1999) underlined the fact that certain methodological issues concerning culture-bound syndromes need to be defined and, to this end, they proposed a research program that made it possible to understand them in their own terms and to determine whether these syndromes could be related to the mental disorders classified by western systems of diagnosis.

The issues that, according to these authors, should be included in research conducted in order to reach an understanding of the holistic nature of culture-bound syndromes are as follows: identifying the nature of the phenomenon, situating the syndrome within the social context, the relation between the syndrome and the psychiatric disorders included in current classifications, and the social and psychiatric history of the syndrome. By following these steps it will be possible to correctly identify the phenomenology and subtypes of the syndrome, the social characteristics of the people who suffer from it and the risk factors, as well as to study the relation with other psychiatric disorders and even other syndromes that are specific to other cultures.

Following these guidelines, the GLDP (APAL, 2004) includes some syndromes that present specifically in Latin American countries and which are not included in the DSM-IV (APA, 1994), such as *atontado* (Tuxtlas, Veracruz, Mexico), *brujería* (Latin America), *colerina* (Distas, Yucatan), *el bla* (Miskitos in Honduras and Nicaragua) and *síndrome de la Nevada* (Peru).

These culture-specific manifestations of the symptoms are determined by beliefs about mental illness that are shared by the group. Such beliefs attempt to explain the causes of the disorder (loss of spiritual strength, loss of the soul) and, therefore, will also determine the popular belief regarding the most effective treatment for it (exorcisms, spells) as well as the person who has to provide that treatment (shaman, medicine man). Thus,

apart from the rational, modern discourse of medicine about disease, there is also a popular, folk or ethnic discourse that attempts to integrate the understanding of morbid processes in a wider, all-embracing conception of disease, life and death. The two discourses often co-exist in apparent harmony, sometimes discussing things with one another and sometimes just coming into conflict. The psychiatrist must understand humans in their world of life, the one where they build their knowledge, otherwise he will understand nothing about his patients or about their illness. (APAL, 2004, p. 17)

It is also known that certain clinical conditions that were thought to be specific to a particular region in fact have a pan-cultural extension. Nevertheless, there have also been reports of certain especially relevant therapeutic and ethnopharmacological peculiarities that are specific to the geographical location in which the disorder takes place (APAL, 2004). Hence, the study of these culture-bound syndromes is crucial to account for some of the issues outlined in this chapter, such as the low rates of usage of mental health services by certain cultural groups and the scant therapeutic compliance in both pharmacological and psychological treatment; it is also important for stimulating research on the confirmation of empirically validated treatments that take into account these and other characteristics of the individual.

## Cultural contributions to DSM-IV

As we have seen above, the growing number of transculturally oriented epidemi-ological studies made it clear that ignoring the influence of cultural factors in (1) psychopathological experience, (2) the manifestation, assessment and course of mental illnesses, and (3) response to treatment, could lead to diagnostic errors and to the appearance of stereotyped ideas about the mental health of certain cultural groups. These results highlighted the urgent need to draw up a set of cultural prin-ciples that regulated the contents of a manual of psychiatric diagnosis, which would have represented an increased understanding of the richness of patients' lives and their worlds, as well as an appreciation of the social burdens that come from ethnic marginalization (Fabrega, 1974; Kleinman, 1986).

Yet, beyond a brief mention in the introductory sections, this cultural approach did not have any special impact during the drafting of the DSM-III or the DSM-III-R (APA, 1980, 1987) and it was not until the fourth edition of the DSM (APA, 1994) was being prepared that the possibility of considering culture in the diagnosis was finally taken seriously (Mezzich, 1996).

It was finally included as a result of work started in 1991, after the Conference on Culture and Psychiatric Diagnosis, which was held under the auspices of the National Institute of Mental Health (NIMH) and the American Psychiatric Association (APA). The main conclusion reached at this conference was the need to identify specific points that enhance the DSM-IV culturally (i.e. in the Introduction to the manual, with cultural considerations pertinent to the various diagnostic categories and the multiaxial schema, and with a glossary of culture-bound syndromes), and the need to confirm the representativeness of the DSM-IV field trial samples, as well as to prepare educative and research materials. To carry out these tasks, 50 experts in cultural psychiatry working in both the clinical and academic fields were chosen to form the Culture and Diagnosis Group (Mezzich, Fabrega & Kleinman, 1992).

Following a great deal of painstaking consultation and revision work carried out between April 1992 and September 1993, the NIMH Culture and Diagnosis Group drew up a first draft of specific cultural proposals, the final version of which is included in the DSM-IV Source Book section on cultural issues (Mezzich *et al.*, 1993).

In 1996, Mezzich *et al.* collected the main cultural proposals, regardless of whether they were included in the DSM-IV or not, with the hope that publishing such information would spur on advances in future systems of psychiatric diagnosis and enrich clinical practice. These proposals were as follows: (1) cultural statement for the introduction to the manual, (2) cultural considerations for various diagnostic categories, (3) cultural annotations for the multiaxial schema, (4) cultural formulation guidelines, and (5) glossary of culture-bound syndromes and idioms of distress (Mezzich *et al.*, 1996).

Multiaxial diagnosis represents a challenging reconceptualization of the diagnostic formulation. As contrasted with the traditional disease entity approach, it involves a schematic and comprehensive statement designed to portray more thoroughly and effectively the patient's condition, to facilitate comprehensive treatment planning, and to maximize prognosis of multiple outcomes. Consequently, cultural factors should be pointedly considered in the development and instrumentation of the various axes, and field trials should address the reliability and validity of the multiaxial system across pertinent ethnic groups and subcultures. Not as a standardized or nomothetic axis but rather as an idiographic or formalized statement, DSM has included for the first time in an official diagnostic system a Cultural Formulation Outline (Mezzich *et al.*, 1993). The components of the DSM-IV Cultural Formulation Outline follow:

A. Cultural identity of the individual
B. Cultural explanations of the individual's illness
C. Cultural factors related to psychosocial environment and levels of functioning

D. Cultural elements of the relationship between the individual and the clinician
E. Overall cultural assessment for diagnosis and care.

From the cultural point of view, this formulation was the main step forward in the DSM-IV, despite the fact that the placement of this Cultural Formulation Outline in the ninth appendix of DSM-IV drastically limits the visibility and accessibility of this development (Mezzich, 1996). We will now go on to examine the repercussions the Cultural Formulation is having on current diagnostic systems.

## Current perspectives in psychiatric diagnosis

The diagnosis is one of the most important key concepts in psychiatry and medicine, because only a good diagnosis will lead to a good treatment. For this reason, from the seventies onwards, the emphasis in psychopathological research has been focused on increasing the reliability of diagnostic concepts in order to achieve the maximum agreement among observers and thus increase the number of effective methods of assessment and intervention.

Three major methodological developments have been cited as being fundamental for increasing the diagnostic reliability in psychiatry in recent years: (a) the use of phenomenological descriptions of disorders; (b) the use of explicit operative criteria for the diagnosis; and (c) the use of multiaxial schemas in the description of the clinical condition, the aim being to capture the components that are critical for the treatment and progression of the patient (Mezzich, 1995).

With regard to the use of explicit operative criteria for the diagnosis, the CIE-10 (World Health Organization, 1997) and the DSM-IV (APA, 1994) have been proposed as universals within the speciality. Nevertheless, in view of the findings from transcultural research, it seems that they are not enough to reflect the idiosyncratic ways of experiencing a disease and the particular clinical needs of certain populations.

Mention should be made at this point of Lain-Entralgo (1982), who pointed out that diagnosis not only involves the identification of diseases (nosological diagnosis) or the distinction between different diseases (differential diagnosis); rather it implies a thorough understanding of what is going on in the mind and body of the person who is seeking clinical healthcare. This must include the particular way an illness is manifested and how each patient goes through a disease, how this affects their familial and social relationships, and the impact it has on their quality of life. And this understanding must be contextualized within the background and culture of each patient in order to make sense. Nevertheless, it has recently been argued that the use of symbols and meanings that are only pertinent to the identity and perspectives of particular patients may lead to the loss of diagnostic validity (Tasman, 2000).

Therefore, in this increasingly multicultural world we live in it is essential to make efforts to accomplish an effective integration of universalism (which facilitates professional communication across the continents) and local realities and needs (which evidence the patient's singularity in his or her particular context) (Mezzich *et al.*, 2003).

It is within this multicultural framework, and thanks to the collaboration among the Diagnostic Assessment and Classification Committees and Sections of the CIE-10 (World Health Organization, 1997), DSM-IV (APA, 1994), the Chinese Classification of Mental Disorders (CCMD-2R) (Chinese Medical Association, 1995) and the Third Cuban Glossary of Psychiatry (GC-3) (Otero, 2000), that a workgroup made up of representative experts from several theoretical approaches and fields of psychiatry from every continent developed the project that was to draw up the International Guidelines for Diagnostic Assessment (IGDA) (Mezzich *et al.*, 2003).

The IGDA project has four fundamental features: (1) it includes the assessment of the psychiatric patient as a whole person, instead of considering them as just carriers of an illness, which means the clinician has to combine scientific competence together with humanistic and ethical aspects in his or her praxis; (2) it covers all the key areas of information (i.e. biological, psychological and social) that are relevant to describing the patient's pathology, dysfunctions and problems, as well as its positive aspects or advantages; (3) it includes basing the diagnostic assessment on an interaction between clinicians, patients and their families, thus facilitating a joint understanding of the patient's clinical condition and an agreement on and monitoring of the care plan; (4) it uses the CIE-10 for the first three axes of its multiaxial formulation (classification of mental disorders, general medical conditions, disabilities and contextual factors) (Mezzich *et al.*, 2003).

One of the most innovating contributions of the diagnostic model proposed in these guidelines is that it combines idiographic elements within a standardized multiaxial system, in contrast to the conventional, reductionist opinions that favor only one of these elements.

The idiographic component of this diagnostic model includes three elements: (a) the perspectives of the clinician; (b) the perspectives of the patients and their families; and (c) the integration of the clinician's perspectives with those of the patient and their family.

Thus, the personalized formulation begins by acknowledging the clinician's, the patient's and (whenever appropriate) the family's perspectives on what is unique, important and meaningful about the patient. The formulation sets out these perspectives and identifies any discrepancies, permitting their resolution and integration into a shared understanding of the case at hand.

At the same time the clinician's perspectives should represent a synthesizing and integrative effort to identify the essential features of the patient's clinical condition and the biological (genetic, molecular and toxic), psychological (psychodynamic, behavioral and cognitive) and social (support and culture) factors that are relevant to that condition. The perspectives of the patient and the family, on the other hand, should cover their understanding of the clinical condition and its contributing factors, the patient's self-image, assets and strengths, and sense of what is meaningful in life. The clinician will use the clinical interview to elicit this information by asking questions such as "What problem brought you here?" "How do you explain what is happening to you?" "How important is it to you?" and "What do you expect the treatment to do for you?" The most important factor for eliciting the patient's and the family's perspectives is the ability to listen well. Learning to listen requires didactic instruction, practice and feedback, together with knowledge of the patient's cultural background.

Integration of the clinician's and the patient's perspectives, essential for a good therapeutic alliance, should be based on an empathetic rapport that reflects mutual respect and interest, and human feeling between the clinician and the patient. The two of them (with the collaboration of the family as needed) should attempt to reach a joint understanding, as far as possible, of the clinical problems and their contextualization, the patient's positive factors, and expectations about restoring and promoting health.

Finally, the clinician, the patient and the family should jointly monitor the progress of care and its outcomes, and also agree on any adjustments that may be necessary.

With regard to the standardized multiaxial assessment, of the score of schemas that have been published (and reviewed by Mezzich, 1979), the ones that are currently most frequently seen are those included in the CIE-10 (World Health Organization, 1997) and the DSM-IV (APA, 1994). Although these systems vary in the number of axes they have, their contents do largely match up: axis I (Clinical diagnoses) of the CIE-10 covers the contents of the first three axes of the DSM-IV; axis II of the CIE-10 assesses the area of disabilities divided into four aspects (personal care, occupational, with the family, and social in general), and corresponds to axis V of the DSM-IV; finally, axis III (Contextual factors) of the CIE-10 essentially matches axis IV of the DSM-IV.

As pointed out earlier, the IGDA utilizes the CIE-10 for the first three axes of its multiaxial formulation. This diagnostic model is structured as follows:

Axis I:     Clinical disorders (mental disorders and general medical conditions)
Axis II:     Disabilities (in personal care, family functioning, social)

Axis III:  Contextual factors (interpersonal, psychosocial and environmental problems)

Axis IV:  Quality of life (patients' own perceptions about the level of their physical and emotional well-being, their functioning, the social support they receive and the fulfillment of their personal and spiritual aspirations)

The domains of this multiaxial formulation should be assessed with sensitivity to the patient's culture. That is to say, identification and rating of the importance of significant problems in health, functioning and social context should be performed bearing in mind the relevant cultural norms and customs.

In conclusion, in these International Guidelines for Diagnostic Assessment from the World Psychiatric Association, the process of clinical assessment is aimed at eliciting the information needed to carry out an integrated diagnostic formulation. This process must be organized in a competent manner in order to obtain reliable, valid information and must be conducted in a climate of respect towards the person being assessed and with a therapeutic purpose. Rather than being just an exercise in taxonomy, a diagnostic assessment represents the first step in the process of clinical care, the fundamental goal of which is to restore and foster the individual's health and to enrich his or her quality of life; taking the patient's cultural surroundings into account is a key aspect in this process (Mezzich *et al.*, 2003).

## Therapeutic response to treatments

Considerations of cultural aspects can offer an alternative framework in which various aspects that may influence the effects of treatment can be identified. With regard to how the patient responds to therapy, some of the arguments used to justify the lack of efficacy of certain treatments for mental disorders have included the elements such as the patient's dissatisfaction, unequal access to medical care or the high costs of such treatments (Wight, Botticello & Aneshensel, 2006; Aneshensel & Phelan, 1999). However, in order to understand this lack of efficacy it is necessary to take into account explanations that derive from, for example, anthropological and transcultural research.

In the context of psychological treatments, cultural differences between the therapist and patient (such as in language, values and expectations) are important determining factors for patient satisfaction and the therapeutic relationship between patient and therapist, which will subsequently determine prospective treatment adherence (Jackson *et al.*, 2007). In a similar way, the use of psychotherapeutic strategies deriving mainly from western theoretical orientation can have limited usefulness in patients from different cultures. Therefore it is generally necessary to modify the existing therapeutic strategies, so that these are compatible to the relevant cultural contexts. (Collazos *et al.*, 2005).

On the other hand, the therapeutic response to pharmacological treatments may be influenced by ethnicity as a result of genetic factors (such as variations in allele frequencies among different ethnic groups) and environmental factors, and/or the interaction between them. In recent years there has been a growing interest in the variations in the pharmacological response to the drugs among different cultural groups (Collazos *et al.*, 2005). In a recent study of the response to antipsychotic treatment in schizophrenia, major ethnic differences were found, indicating that cross-ethnic factors such as diet, nutritional status, body mass and substance use could be important, as well as genetically determined ethno-specific pharmacokinetic and pharmacodynamic differences (Emsley, Roberts, Rataemane *et al.*, 2002).

## Conclusion

To finish on the subject of the importance that culture has in psychopathology, future studies into culture and psychopathology should develop and include measures capable of directly assessing cultural factors. If psychopathological research fails to take cultural aspects into account, variations in people's behavior, beliefs and experience that are considered to be completely normal in their source culture may be (wrongly) interpreted as being of a psychopathological nature. In Latin America psychotropic plants are consumed in sacred rites and this should not be confused with problems of addiction or the recreational use of drugs, an example being the consumption of coca leaves in the plateaus of Peru and Bolivia. Likewise, in certain rural areas there are a number of zoophilias that are culturally tolerated and that do not fulfill the strict criteria of a mental or developmental disorder (APAL, 2004).

Furthermore, the predictive model drawn up by Agbayani-Siewert *et al.* (1999) requires these measures to be culturally appropriate and relevant because current epidemiological research uses western concepts to explain the ways psychopathological manifestations are expressed, help-seeking behaviors, the use of services and the application of treatments, and they are unable to represent the experiences of some groups.

Within the area of biological treatments it is especially important to analyze the "non-pharmacological factors" of psychopharmacology, which include the fact that prescription patterns vary from one ethnic group to another: colored patients in the United States receive greater doses of neuroleptic drugs and injectable or depot forms are more frequent than oral medication (Alarcón, 2005); how side effects are perceived and reported are strongly affected by the patient's (culturally determined) beliefs and perspectives (Lin, Poland & Nakasaki, 1993). Some studies show that the doses of certain psychotropic agents that are required to be effective seem to be lower in cultures that promote interdependence and social adaptation (Murphy, 1969). Lastly, levels of stress, the quality and quantity of social support and interpersonal styles are cultural factors that exert a decisive influence on the response to psychotropic agents.

Therefore, without neglecting the biological and psychological components in accounting for psychopathological behaviors, we should turn our attention away from the individual and focus on society so as to see mental illness as a process involving social interaction and reaction. This perspective represents a "person-in-environment" model that integrates biological, psychological, sociostructural and cultural factors (Agbayani-Siewert *et al.*, 1999), thus allowing a comprehensive diagnosis to be made.

It is essential to make efforts to achieve an effective integration of universalism (which facilitates professional communication across the continents) and local realities and needs (which evidence the patient's singularity in his or her particular context). The standardized diagnostic formula (CIE-10, DSM-IV) must therefore be combined with an idiographic, or personalized, diagnostic formulation that reflects the individuality and singularity of each patient's personal experience. At the nomothetic level, a multiaxial diagnostic formulation is recommended. For the personalized formulation, an integration of the perspectives of the clinician, the patient and the family should be presented in natural language (Mezzich *et al.*, 2003).

## REFERENCES

Adebimpe, V. R. (1994). Race, racism, and epidemiological surveys. *Hosp. Community Psychiatry*, **45**(1), 27–31.

Adebimpe, V. R., Chu, C. & Klein, H. E. (1982). Racial and geographic differences in the psychopathology of schizophrenia. *Am. J. Psychiatry*, **139**(7), 888–91.

Agbayani-Siewert, P., Takeuchi D. & Pangan, R. (1999). Mental illness in a multicultural context. In C. Aneshensel and J. Phelann, eds., *Handbook of the Sociology of Mental Health*. New York: Kluwer Academic/Plenum Publishers, pp. 19–36.

Alarcón, R. D. (2005). Psiquiatría cultural. In J. V. Vallejo and C. Leal, eds., *Tratado de Psiquiatría*, Vol. II. Barcelona: Ars Médica, pp. 2244–58.

Alegria, M., Takeuchi, D., Canino, G. *et al.* (2004). Considering context, place and culture: The National Latino and Asian American Study. *Int. J. Methods Psychiatr. Res.*, **13**(4), 208–20.

Allen, T. (1992). Taking culture seriously. In T. Allen and A. Thomas, eds., *Poverty and Development in the 1990s*. Oxford: Oxford University Press.

American Psychiatric Association [APA] (1980). *Diagnostic and Statistical Manual of Mental Disorders*, 3rd edn. (DSM-III). Washington, DC: APA Press.

American Psychiatric Association [APA] (1987). *Diagnostic and Statistical Manual of Mental Disorders*, 3rd edn., Revised (DSM-III-R). Washington, DC: APA Press.

American Psychiatric Association [APA] (1994). *Diagnostic and Statistical Manual of Mental Disorders*, 4th edn. (DSM-IV). Washington, DC: APA Press.

Aneshensel, C. S. & Phelan, J. C. (1999). *Handbook of the Sociology of Mental Health.* New York: Kluwer Academic/Plenum Publishers.

Asociación Psiquiátrica de América Latina (Latin American Psychiatric Association) [APAL] (2004). *Guía Latinoamericana de Diagnóstico Psiquiátrico* (*Latin American Guide for Psychiatric Diagnosis*) [GLADP]. Mexico: Universidad de Guadalajara.

Bell, C. & Mehta, H. (1980). The misdiagnosis of black patients with manic depressive illness. *J. Natl. Med. Assoc.,* **72**(2), 141–5.

Berreman, G. (1991). The Brahminical view of caste. In D. Gupta (ed.), *Social Stratification.* Delhi: OUP, pp. 84–92.

Berry, J. W. (1997). Immigration, acculturation, and adaptation. *Applied Psychology: An International Review,* **46**(1), 5–34.

Berry, J. W. (2006). Acculturative stress. In P. T. P. Wong & L. C. J. Wong, eds., *Handbook of Multicultural Perspectives on Stress and Coping.* Dallas, TX: Spring Publications, pp. 287–98.

Berry, J. W., Phinney, J. S., Sam, D. L. & Vedder, P. (2006). Immigrant youth: acculturation, identity, and adaptation. *Applied Psychology: An International Review,* **55**(3), 303–32.

Bevis, W. M. (1921). Psychological traits of the Southern Negro with observations as to some of his psychoses. *Am. J. Psychiatry,* **1**, 69–78.

Blackledge, A. (2003). Imagining a monocultural community: racialization of cultural practice in educational discourse. *J. Language, Identity, and Education,* **2**(4), 331–47.

Cacioppo, J. T. & Berntson, G. G. (1992). Social psychological contributions to the decade of the brain: doctrine of multilevel analysis. *Am. Psychol.,* **47**(8), 1019–28.

Cacioppo, J. T. & Berntson, G. G. (2006). A bridge linking social psychology and the neurosciences. In P. A. M. Van Lange, ed., *Bridging Social Psychology: Benefits of Transdisciplinary Approaches.* Mahwah, NJ: Lawrence Erlbaum Associates Publishers, pp. 91–6.

Cameron, J. E. & Lalonde, R. N. (1994). Self, ethnicity, and social group memberships in two generations of Italian Canadians. *Pers. Soc. Psychol. Bull.,* **20**(5), 514–20.

Chang, D. (2002). *Understanding the Rates and Distribution of Mental Disorders. Asian American Mental Health: Assessment Theories and Methods.* New York: Kluwer Academic/Plenum Publishers, pp. 9–27.

Cheng, C., Lee, F. & Benet-Martínez, V. (2006). Assimilation and contrast effects in cultural frame switching: bicultural identity integration and valence of cultural cues. *J. Cross Cult. Psychol.,* **37**(6), 742–60.

Cheung, F. M. (1989). The indigenization of neurasthenia in Hong Kong. *Cult. Med. Psychiatry,* **13**, 227–41.

Cheung, F. M. & Bernard, W. (1982). Situational variations of help-seeking behavior among Chinese patients. *Compr. Psychiatry,* **23**(3), 252–62.

Chinese Medical Association (1995). *Chinese Classification of Mental Disorders,* 2nd edn., revised. Nanjing, China: Dong Nan University Press.

Collazos, F., Achotegui, J., Caballero, L. & Casas, M. (2005). Emigración y psicopatología. In J. V. Vallejo and C. Leal, eds., *Tratado de Psiquiatría* (vol. II). Barcelona: Ars Médica, pp. 2259–72.

Eaton, J. W. & Weil, R. J. (1955). *Culture and Mental Disorders.* New York, NY: Free Press.

Emsley, R. A., Roberts, M. C., Rataemane, S. *et al.* (2002). Ethnicity and treatment response in schizophrenia: a comparison of 3 ethnic groups. *J. Clin. Psychiatry*, **63**(1), 9–14.

Fábrega, H. (1995). Cultural challenges to the psychiatric enterprise. *Compr. Psychiatry*, **36**(5), 377–83.

Fabrega, H. Jr. (1974). *Disease and Social Behavior: An Interdisciplinary Perspective.* Cambridge, MA: MIT Press.

Guarnaccia, P. J. N. & Rogler, L. H. (1999). Research on culture-bound syndromes: new directions. *Am. J. Psychiatry,* **156**(9), 1322–7.

Guarnaccia, P. J., Angel, R. & Worobey , J. L. (1989). The factor structure of the CES-D in the Hispanic Health and Nutrition Examination Survey: the influences of ethnicity, gender, and language. *Soc. Sci. Med.,* **29**(1), 85–94.

Hofstede, G. (1980). *Culture's Consequences: International Differences in Work-Related Values.* Beverly Hills, CA: Sage.

Jackson, J. S., Neighbors, H. W., Torres, M. *et al.* (2007). Use of mental health services and subjective satisfaction with treatment among Black Caribbean immigrants: results from the National Survey of American Life. *Am. J. Public Health,* **97**(1), 60–7.

Kimmich, R. A. (1960). Ethnic aspects of schizophrenia in Hawaii. *Psychiatry,* **23**, 97–102.

Kitano, H. H. L. (1962). Changing achievement patterns of the Japanese in the United States. *J. Soc. Psychol.,* **58**(2), 257–64.

Kleinman, A. M. (1977). Depression, somatization and the new cross-cultural psychiatry. *Soc. Sci. Med.,* **11**(1), 3–10.

Kleinman, A. M. (1986). *Social Origins of Distress and Disease.* New Haven, CT: Yale University Press.

Kleinman, A. M. (1988). A window on mental health in China. *Am. Sci.,* **76**(1), 22–7.

Lain-Entralgo, P. (1982). *El diagnóstico médico* (Medical diagnosis). Barcelona: Salvat.

Lin, K-M., Poland, R. E. & Nakasaki, G. (1993). *Psychopharmacology and Psychobiology of Ethnicity.* Washington, DC : APA.

Lin, T. (1982). Culture and psychiatry: a Chinese perspective. *Aust. N. Z. J. Psychiatry,* **16**(4), 235–45.

López, S. R & Guarnaccia, P. J. (2005). In J. E. Maddux and B. A. Winstead, eds., *Psychopathology: Foundations for a Contemporary Understanding.* Mahwah, NJ: Lawrence Erlbaum Associates Publishers, pp. 19–37.

MacLachlan, M. (1997). *Culture and Health.* Chichester, England: John Wiley and Sons, Inc.

Malgady, R. G., Rogler, L. H. & Cortes, D. E. (1996). Cultural expression of psychiatric symptoms: idioms of anger among Puerto Ricans. *Psychol. Assess.,* **8**, 265–8.

Marsella, A. J. (1988). Cross-cultural research on severe mental disorders: issues and findings. *Acta Psychiatr. Scand.,* **78**(344 Suppl), 7–22.

Marsella, A. J., Kinzie, D. & Gordon, P. (1973). Ethnic variations in the expression of depression. *J. Cross Cult. Psychol.,* **4**(4), 435–58.

Mezzich, J. E. (1979). Patterns and issues in multiaxial psychiatric diagnosis. *Psychol. Med.*, **9**(1) 125–7.

Mezzich, J. E. (1995). Cultural formulation and comprehensive diagnosis: clinical and research perspectives. *Psychiatr. Clin. North Am.*, **18**, 649–57.

Mezzich, J. E. (1996). Culture and multiaxial diagnosis. In J. E. Mezzich, A. Kleinman, H. Fabrega and D. L. Parron, eds., *Culture and Psychiatric Diagnosis. A DSM-IV Perspective*. Washington, DC: APA Press, pp. 327–34.

Mezzich, J. E., Fabrega, H. & Kleinman, A. (1992). Cultural validity and DSM-IV (editorial). *J. Nerv. Ment. Dis.*, **180**, 4.

Mezzich, J. E., Kleinman, A., Fábrega, H. *et al.* (eds.) (1993). Revised cultural proposals for DSM-IV. Working document submitted to the DSM-IV Task Force by the NIMH-sponsored Group on Culture and Diagnosis.

Mezzich, J. E., Kleinman, A. E., Fabrega, H. J. E. & Parron, D. L. E. (1996). *Culture and Psychiatric Diagnosis: A DSM-IV Perspective*. Washington, DC: American Psychiatric Press, Inc.

Mezzich, J. E., Lewis-Fernández, R. & Ruipérez, M. A. (2003). The cultural framework of psychiatric disorders. In A. Tasman, J. Kay and J. A. Lieberman, eds., *Psychiatry*, 2nd edn. London: John Wiley & Sons, pp. 645–55.

Mezzich, J. E., Berganza, C. E., von Cranach, M. *et al.* (2003). Essentials of the WPA International Guidelines for Diagnostic Assessment (IGDA). *Br. J. Psychiatry. Suppl.* **45**.

Ming-Yuan, Z. (1989). The diagnosis and phenomenology of neurasthenia: a Shanghai study. *Cult. Med. Psychiatry,* **13**(2), 147–61.

Murphy, H. B. (1969). Ethnic variations in drug response: results of an international survey. *Transcultural Psychiatric Res.*, **6**, 5–23.

Otero, A. A. (ed.) (2000). *Tercer Glosario Cubano de Psiquiatría* (Third Cuban Glossary of Psychiatry). Havana, Cuba: Hospital Psiquiátrico de La Habana.

Rubel, A. J. (1964). The study of Latino folk illnesses. *Med. Anthropol.*, **15**(2), 209–13.

Sam, D. L., Vedder, P., Ward, C. & Horenczyk, G. (2006). Psychological and sociocultural adaptation of immigrant youth. In J. W. Berry, J. S. Phinney, D. L. Sam and P. Vedder, eds., *Immigrant Youth in Cultural Transition: Acculturation, Identity, and Adaptation Across National Contexts*. Mahwah, NJ: Lawrence Erlbaum Associates Publishers, pp. 117–41.

Searle, W. & Ward, C. (1990). The prediction of psychological and sociocultural adjustment during cross-cultural transitions. *Intl. J. Intercultural Relations,* **14**(4), 449–64.

Sue, D. W. & Kirk, B. A. (1975). Asian-Americans: use of counseling and psychiatric services on a college campus. *J. Counseling Psychology,* **22**(1), 84–6.

Szapocznik, J. & Kurtines, W. M. (1993). Family psychology and cultural diversity: opportunities for theory, research, and application. *Am. Psychol.*, **48**(4), 400–7.

Tasman, A. (2000). Lost in the DSM-IV checklist: empathy, meaning, and the doctor–patient relationship. Presidential address, Proceedings of the 153rd Annual Meeting of the American Psychiatric Association, Chicago, IL.

Torrey, E. F. (1995). Prevalence of psychosis among the Hutterites: a reanalysis of the 1950–53 study. *Schizophr. Res.*, **16**(2), 167–70.

Triandis, H. C. (1993). Collectivism and individualism as cultural syndromes. *Cross-Cultural Research: The Journal of Comparative Social Science,* **27**(3–4), 155–80.

Tseng, W-S. (1975). The nature of somatic complaints among psychiatric patients: the Chinese case. *Compr. Psychiatry,* **16**(3), 237–45.

Ward, C. (1996). Acculturation. In Landis, D. and Bhagat, R. S., eds., *Handbook of Intercultural Training,* 2nd edn. Thousand Oaks, CA: Sage Publications, pp. 124–47.

Ward, C. & Kennedy, A. (1999). The measurement of sociocultural adaptation. *Intl. J. Intercultural Relations,* **23**(4), 659–77.

Westen, D. (2004). Culture on the ground and in the brain. *PsycCRITIQUES.* American Psychological Association.

Wight, R. G., Botticello, A. L. & Aneshensel, C. S. (2006). Socioeconomic context, social support, and adolescent mental health: a multilevel investigation. *J. Youth and Adolescence,* **35**(1), 115–26.

Williams, D. H. (1986). The epidemiology of mental illness in Afro-Americans. *Hosp. Community Psychiatry,* **37**(1), 42–9.

Williams, D. R., Yu, Y. & Jackson, J. S. (1997). Racial differences in physical and mental health: socio-economic status, stress and discrimination. *Journal of Health Psychology,* **2**(3), 335–51.

World Health Organization (1997). *Multiaxial Presentation of ICD-10 for use in Adult Psychiatry.* Cambridge, UK: Cambridge University Press.

Yamamoto, J., James, Q. C. & Palley, N. (1968). Cultural problems in psychiatric therapy. *Arch. Gen. Psychiatry,* **19**(1), 45–9.

Zhang, D. (1995). Depression and culture: a Chinese perspective. *Can. J. Counselling,* **29**, 227–33.

**3**

# Culture and ethnicity in psychopharmacotherapy

Keh-Ming Lin, Chia-Hui Chen, Shu-Han Yu,
and Sheng-Chang Wang

## Introduction

The use of psychiatric medication has transcended geographic, cultural, and ethnic boundaries during the past several decades (Lin, Poland *et al.*, 1993; Lin & Cheung, 1999; Lin & Smith, 2000). Within a few years of their discovery, modern psychotropics have achieved worldwide acceptance as the mainstay for the treatment of the mentally ill (Lin, Poland *et al.*, 1993; Ng, Lin *et al.*, 2005). This notwithstanding, until most recently, clinicians and researchers have paid little attention to potential influences of ethnic and cultural factors on pharmacotherapeutic responses. With a few prominent exceptions, practically all psychiatric medications have been developed and tested in North America and Western Europe, and often, on "young, white males." In addition, since these research efforts usually aim at defining what are "typical" that can be generalized, variations in responses are often regarded as "noises" and consequently ignored. Therefore, although substantial differences in psychotropic responses have been repeatedly observed and documented in the literature, such information has not been widely disseminated, and our knowledge in this regard is still sparse and unsystematic. Treatment decisions are generally not individualized; choice of medication and dosing routines are largely based on "trial and error" practices rather than on rational principles.

In contrast, recent literature clearly demonstrates that ethnicity and culture powerfully determine individuals' pharmacological responses (Lin & Poland, 1995). These responses are shaped simultaneously by genetic and environmental factors. On the genetic side, genetic polymorphisms with functional significance have been identified in most genes encoding drug metabolizing enzymes as well as the putative targets of pharmaceutical agents (e.g., neurotransmitter receptors and transporters). Patterns of these genetic polymorphisms often vary substantially across

*Ethno-psychopharmacology: Advances in Current Practice*, eds. C. H. Ng, K.-M. Lin, B. S. Singh and E. Y. K. Chiu. Published by Cambridge University Press. © C. H. Ng, K.-M. Lin, B. S. Singh and E. Y. K. Chiu 2008.

ethnic groups, resulting in variations in the activities of proteins controlling both the metabolism and the effects of pharmacotherapeutic agents. In addition, the expressions of these genes are often significantly modified by a large number of environmental factors, including diet and exposure to various substances (e.g., tobacco and herbal preparations).

Of even greater importance, the success of any therapy, including pharmacotherapy, depends on the relationship between patient and therapist. The nature and quality of the interaction between the clinician and the patient, flavored by both of their cultural backgrounds, values, attitudes, and expectations, serve as the backdrop against which drugs work, or fail to work. Attention to and successful management of transference and counter-transference are key to the success of not only psychotherapy, but also pharmacotherapy. The importance of culture in this respect cannot be disregarded.

The literature documenting cultural and ethnic influences on pharmacological responses has been reviewed and commented by various authors in recent years. These data came from reports derived from various sources and studies utilizing divergent designs, including surveys of drug utilization and dosing patterns, case reports, chart reviews, drug pharmacokinetics/pharmacodynamics, and prospective treatment studies. Findings from these studies convincingly demonstrate that significant cross-ethnic drug response variations exist in practically all classes of medications, especially with regard to psychotropics, cardiovascular, and antineoplastic medications. For example, a series of studies demonstrated that, as compared to their Caucasian counterparts, Asians are often successfully treated with lower dosages of haloperidol and other neuroleptics in hospitalized inpatients (Lin, Poland *et al.*, 1988; Lin, Poland *et al.*, 1993). When given comparable doses of medication, Asian patients with schizophrenia and Asian normal volunteers exhibited plasma haloperidol concentrations that were approximately 50% greater than their Caucasian counterparts (see Figure 3.1).

At the same time, the study also showed a greater prolactin response to haloperidol in Asians than Caucasians. When receiving comparable doses of intramuscular (IM) haloperidol, Asian patients had higher plasma prolactin concentrations than their Caucasian counterparts (Lin, Poland *et al.*, 1988). This difference remained statistically significant after controlling for ethnic variations in plasma haloperidol concentrations. In a subsequent clinical treatment study, Asian patients with schizophrenia responded optimally to significantly lower plasma haloperidol concentrations as compared to their Caucasian counterparts (Lin, Poland *et al.*, 1989). These data, together with many other studies, suggested that both pharmacokinetic and pharmacodynamic mechanisms were responsible for previous observations of Asians requiring lower doses of neuroleptics for similar therapeutic responses. It is now clear that both processes are controlled by genetic factors, and that the expression of genes are at the same time strongly influenced by environmental

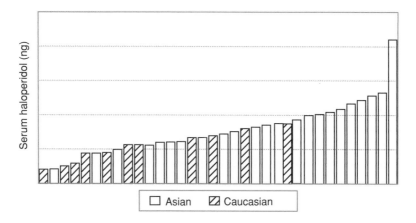

Figure 3.1    Maximal haloperidol concentration after 0.5 mg intramuscular haloperidol

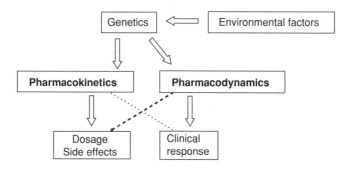

Figure 3.2    Factors determining pharmacological response

factors. Thus, as is true in most biological processes, drug metabolism and drug responses are determined by gene–environmental interactions. With this understanding, the significance of both ethnicity and culture in determining drug response becomes self evident (see Figure 3.2).

## Drug-metabolizing enzymes

A limited number of enzymes are involved in the biotransformation of all drugs, including psychotropics. Among the drug-metabolizing enzymes, the most important ones are those belonging to the cytochrome P 450 system (Lin, Smith *et al.*, 2003). Most psychotropics are metabolized by one or more of the following four cytochrome enzymes: CYP2D6, CYP3A4, CYP1A2, and CYP2C19. Genetic differences in the genes controlling these enzymes (genetic polymorphisms) lead to extremely large variations in their activities within and between populations (Lin & Poland, 1995). CYP2D6 is the most dramatic example, with more than

50 mutations, some of them inactivate, impair, or accelerate its function (Daly, Brockmoller *et al.*, 1996). Most of these mutant alleles are to a large extent ethnically specific. For example, *CYP2D6\*4*, which produces defective proteins is found in approximately 25% of Caucasians, but is rarely seen in other ethnic groups. This mutation is mainly responsible for the high rate of poor metabolizers (PM) in Caucasians (5–9%), who are expected to be inefficient in metabolizing CYP2D6 substrates, such as risperidone and paroxetine. Instead of *CYP2D6\*4*, high frequencies of *CYP2D6\*17* (Masimirembwa & Hasler, 1997; Leathart, London *et al.*, 1998) and *CYP2D6\*10* (Wang, Huang *et al.*, 1993; Dahl, Yue *et al.* 1995; Roh, Dahl *et al.*, 1996; Liou, Lin *et al.*, 2006) were found among those of African and Asian origins, respectively. Both of these alleles are associated with lower enzyme activities and slower metabolism of CYP2D6 substrates. "Slow" metabolizers are likely to develop higher plasma concentrations and require lower therapeutic doses. The higher frequency of these less active CYP2D6 alleles in Africans and Asians may explain the lower therapeutic dose ranges of neuroleptics and antidepressants observed in Asians and lower doses of tricyclic antidepressants needed in African Americans (Lin & Poland, 1995). Our recent study showed that Mexican Americans had very low rates of these "deficient" mutations, leading to significantly higher overall CYP2D6 activity in this ethnic background (Mendoza, Wan *et al.*, 2001).

In addition, CYP2D6 is unique because the gene is often duplicated or multiplied (up to 13 copies). Those with these duplicated or multiple genes have more enzymes and higher enzyme activity, and are called "ultra-rapid" metabolizers (UM). Ultra-rapid metabolizers are found in 1% of Swedish, 5% of Spaniards (White Americans are in between these two figures), 19% of Arabics, and 29% of Ethiopians. Patients who are UM may fail to respond to usual doses of medications metabolized by CYP2D6, since their blood level of medication will usually be below therapeutic range unless treated with excessively high doses of the same drugs (Lin, Smith *et al.*, 2003). Patients who were UM were regarded as non-compliant in previous reports because they did not show any evidence of drug effect while given standard doses of medications (Aklillu, Persson *et al.*, 1996). This may be a particularly important issue for Ethiopians since one third of Ethiopians genotyped were UMs, and therefore possibly needed higher doses of medicines whose biotransformation are mediated by CYP2D6, in order to achieve therapeutic response.

CYP2C19 is another example of the existence of both cross-ethnic and inter-individual variations in drug metabolism. This enzyme is involved in the metabolism of many psychotropics such as diazepam and tertiary tricyclic antidepressants, as well as one of the selective serotonin re-uptake inhibitors (SSRIs), citalopram. Using S-mephenytoin as the probe, previous studies showed that up to 20% of East Asians (Chinese, Japanese, and Koreans) are PMs, when only 3–5%

of Caucasians are (Xie, Stein *et al.*, 1999). Since the gene encoding the enzyme had been identified and sequenced, it was reported that such enzyme deficiency is mostly caused by two unique polymorphisms, CYP2C19*2 and CYP2C19*3. While CYP2C19*2 can be found in all ethnic groups, CYP2C19*3 was seen only in those with Eastern Asian origins. The presence of CYP2C19*3 and a higher rate of CYP2C19*2 may be responsible for the higher rate of PMs among Asians. This explains why Asians generally have increased sensitivity to drugs such as diazepam and other substrates of CYP2C19 (de Morais, Wilkinson *et al.*, 1994; Goldstein, Ishizaki *et al.*, 1997).

## Diet and its effect on P450 enzymes

Dietary habits affect pharmacokinetics as they change the body's ability to absorb, distribute, and metabolize medications. A high-protein diet, for example, has been shown to enhance drug metabolism through increased oxidation and conjugation. A high-protein diet accelerates the metabolism of drugs such as antipyrine and theophyllines and a high-carbohydrate diet appears to have the opposite effect (Branch, Salih *et al.*, 1978; Fraser, Mucklow *et al.*, 1979; Anderson & Kappas, 1991). In addition to the "macronutrients" (i.e., proportion of carbohydrates, proteins, and fat in the diet), numerous "micronutrients" also exert major effects on the expression of many drug-metabolizing enzymes. For example, CYP1A2 is inducible by charbroiled beef and cruciferous vegetables, and certain citrus fruits and plant products, such as grapefruits and corn, potently inhibit CYP3A4 (Fuhr, Klittich *et al.*, 1993; Oesterheld and Kallepalli, 1997).

A series of studies conducted in the 1970s clearly highlight the importance of culture and cultural change in determining drug metabolism. Conducted among Sudanese and South Asians before and after their migration to England, these studies showed a substantially slower rate of metabolism of some of the CYP1A2 substrates, such as antipyrine and clomipramine, among these "non-Westerners" as compared to their British White counterparts. Once they immigrated to London and took on new dietary habits, these immigrants' metabolic profiles for CYP1A2 substrates became indistinguishable from the "native" Westerners' (Allen, Rack *et al.*, 1977).

CYP3A4 is highly inducible by a large variety of commonly prescribed and utilized synthetic drugs (e.g., carbamazepine) and plant products (e.g., St. John's wort) (Roby, Anderson *et al.*, 2000), and at the same time also is potently inhibited by various other medications (e.g., terfenadine and ketoconazole) (Jurima-Romet, Crawford *et al.*, 1994) as well as common foodstuffs (e.g., grapefruit juice) (Oesterheld & Kallepalli, 1997). Since individual and ethnic/cultural groups vary dramatically in their exposure to these inducers and inhibitors, it stands to reason that there should be significant variations in the expression of this enzyme, which then should be translated into differences in the metabolism and effects of psychotropics and other medications.

## Smoking and its effect on P450 enzymes

Compared to those without psychiatric disorders, psychiatric patients are significantly more likely to be addicted to nicotine, and also are more likely to become heavier smokers (Lohr & Flynn, 1992; Kelly & McCreadie, 1999; Beratis, Katrivanou *et al.*, 2001). The heavier exposure to tobacco carries with it significant health risk for this vulnerable population that has not been adequately addressed. In addition, even less known is the fact that exposure to tobacco often significantly alters the pharmacokinetics of psychotropics (and other medications), resulting in changes in dosing requirements, side effect profiles, and ultimately patients' response to pharmacotherapy. Polycyclic aromatic hydrocarbons (PAHs) present in cigarette smoke induce several hepatic cytochrome P450 (CYP) isozymes, including CYP1A2 and CYP2E1 (Zevin & Benowitz, 1999). Whereas the induction of CYP2E1 has been implicated in cancer risks associated with smoking (Le Marchand, Sivaraman *et al.*, 1998; Choi, Lee *et al.*, 2003) CYP1A2 induction has been identified as the main reason for the reduction of the plasma concentrations of antidepressants (e.g., imipramine, clomipramine, fluvoxamine, and trazodone), antipsychotics (e.g., chlorpromazine, clozapine, tiotixene, fluphenazine, haloperidol, and olanzapine), and anxiolytics (e.g., alprazolam, lorazepam, oxazepam, diazepam, and demethyl-diazepam). Surprisingly, carbamazepine appears to be minimally affected by cigarette smoking although it has been shown to be a substrate of as well as a potent inducer for CYP1A2. Perhaps this is because hepatic enzymes are at the same time stimulated by the autoinductive properties of this unique medication. Taken together, it is clear that cigarette smoking affects the pharmacokinetic of a large number of psychotropic drugs. Separately, it could also alter drug response via pharmacodynamic mechanisms (Miller, 1989; Schein, 1995). It is thus crucial that clinicians consider smoking as an important factor in prescribing these medications (Zevin & Benowitz, 1999).

## Genetic polymorphisms in gene encoding receptors, transporters, or other therapeutic targets

Although we must await further clarification, a large number of genes have already been identified to exert major influences on therapeutic targets' response to psychotropics (Schildkraut, Kopin *et al.*, 1995). These include genes encoding transporters and receptors of key neurotransmitters believed to be involved in mediating the clinical effects (therapeutic as well as toxic) of most commonly used psychotherapeutic agents. Genes controlling the biosynthesis and catabolism of these neurotransmitters also have been extensively studied. Most of these genes have been found to be polymorphic, and the patterns of these polymorphisms also typically vary significantly across ethnicity. One example is the most extensively studied gene in this regard, namely, the serotonin transporter (5-HTT).

Responsible for the re-uptake of serotonin back to the presynaptic neuron, the 5-HTT is a prime target of most antidepressants whose demonstrated efficacy supports the thesis that 5-HTT indeed plays a crucial role in the pathogenesis of depression, as well as in mediating the effect of antidepressants. A functional insertion/deletion polymorphism in the promoter region of the 5-HTT gene has been shown to modulate its transcription, resulting in differential 5-HTT expression and 5HT cellular uptake (Greenberg, McMahon *et al.*, 1998). Hariri *et al.* reported that subjects who are homozygotic for the *l* allele for HTTLPR showed less fear and anxiety-related behaviors and exhibited less amygdala neuronal activity as assessed by functional MRI, in response to fearful stimuli (Hariri & Weinberger 2003). Of note, the prevalence of the *l* allele varies substantially across ethnic groups, ranging from approximately 70% among populations with sub-Saharan African origin to 30% among East Asians (Gelernter, Kranzler *et al.*, 1997).

The relationship between HTTLPR polymorphisms and antidepressant response has been intriguing. Since 1998, at least five studies conducted in Italy and North America (with predominantly Caucasian patient populations), as well as one from Taiwan, showed that the 5-HTTLPR *l* allele is associated with better or more rapid SSRI response (Smeraldi, Zanardi *et al.*, 1998; Pollock, Ferrell *et al.*, 2000; Zanardi, Serretti *et al.*, 2001; Rausch, Johnson *et al.*, 2002; Yu, Tsai *et al.*, 2002; Arias, Catalan *et al.*, 2003). Two recent studies also implicate the 5HTTLPR *s* allele in SSRI-emergent adverse effects. In contrast, two of three studies conducted in Asia found that the *s* allele was predictive of better SSRI response (Yoshida, Ito *et al.*, 2002; Kim, Lim *et al.*, 2006). Although the mechanism(s) responsible for such cross-ethnic discrepancies in the effect of the HTTLPR polymorphisms remain unclear, they do serve to highlight the importance of taking ethnicity into consideration in designing pharmacogenetic and other genetic studies.

## Non-biologic factors that affect drug response

We have thus far focused on the biological factors that affect drug responses but recovery from illness often takes place in the context of interactions among individuals. In these interactions, both patient and clinician bring their own knowledge, predispositions, values, priorities, modes of thinking, and belief systems into play. Within this transaction, issues such as patient compliance, "expectation effect" (including the placebo effect), clinician ideology, and past experiences impact drug responses (Lin, Elwyn *et al.*, 2004). These "non-biological" factors, which are in a large part shaped by that culture, powerfully determine the success or failure of any pharmacological treatment, regardless of drug receptor specificity or drug potency.

## Conclusion

As is apparent from the literature reviewed above, that culture and ethnicity are powerful determinants of an individual's response to psychopharmacotherapy. Progress in this regard will vastly improve our current practice in using medications. However, it is necessary to remember that there are often very substantial inter-individual variations within any defined cultural or ethnic group, and that ethnic variations in pharmacological responses should not be interpreted stereotypically.

It is likely that progress in pharmacogenomics will eventually lead to specific clinical applications useful for clinicians to guide their decisions in terms of the choice of psychotropics, strategies for titration, as well as the prediction of likely side effects. These developments should result in the formulation of treatment strategies that are not only more effective but also more cost-effective than "traditional" approaches. Together, these exciting new developments should help to make psychopharmacotherapy increasingly more rational, evidence based, and effective. In addition, the progress in pharmacogenetics might also stimulate research on "non-biological" issues such as cultural influences on adherence and other factors that determine patients' perception and action, which in turn contribute towards their sense of satisfaction and benefit from antidepressant treatment. With such an integrative approach, we would be best able to define elements for optimal pharmacotherapeutic practices that would take both cultural and biological diversity into consideration and tailor treatment to individual characteristics rather than relying on generalized guidelines.

## REFERENCES

Aklillu, E. , Persson, I. *et al.* (1996). Frequent distribution of ultrarapid metabolizers of debrisoquine in an Ethiopian population carrying duplicated and multiduplicated functional CYP2D6 alleles. *J. Pharmacol. Exp. Ther.*, **278**(1), 441–6.

Allen, J. J. , Rack, P. H. *et al.* (1977). Differences in the effects of clomipramine on English and Asian volunteers. Preliminary report on a pilot study. *Postgrad. Med. J.*, **53**(4), 79–86.

Anderson, K. E. & Kappas A. (1991). Dietary regulation of cytochrome P450. *Annu. Rev. Nutr.*, **11**, 141–67.

Arias, B., Catalan, R. *et al.* (2003). 5-HTTLPR polymorphism of the serotonin transporter gene predicts non-remission in major depression patients treated with citalopram in a 12-weeks follow up study. *J. Clin. Psychopharmacol.*, **23**(6), 563–7.

Beratis, S. , Katrivanou, A. *et al.* (2001). Factors affecting smoking in schizophrenia. *Compr. Psychiatry*, **42**(5), 393–402.

Branch, R. A. , Salih, S. Y. *et al.* (1978). Racial differences in drug metabolizing ability: a study with antipyrine in the Sudan. *Clin. Pharmacol. Ther.*, **24**(3), 283–6.

Choi, J. Y. , Lee, K. M. *et al.* (2003). CYP2E1 and NQO1 genotypes, smoking and bladder cancer. *Pharmacogenetics*, **13**(6), 349–55.

Dahl, M. L. , Yue, Q. Y. *et al.* (1995). Genetic analysis of the CYP2D locus in relation to debrisoquine hydroxylation capacity in Korean, Japanese and Chinese subjects. *Pharmacogenetics*, **5**(3), 159–64.

Daly, A. K. , Brockmoller, J. *et al.* (1996). Nomenclature for human CYP2D6 alleles. *Pharmacogenetics*, **6**(3), 193–201.

de Morais, S. M. , Wilkinson, G. R. *et al.* (1994). The major genetic defect responsible for the polymorphism of S-mephenytoin metabolism in humans. *J. Biol. Chem.*, **269**(22), 15419–22.

Fraser, H. S. , Mucklow, J. C. *et al.* (1979). Environmental factors affecting antipyrine metabolism in London factory and office workers. *Br. J. Clin. Pharmacol.*, **7**(3), 237–43.

Fuhr, U. , Klittich, K. *et al.* (1993). Inhibitory effect of grapefruit juice and its bitter principal, naringenin, on CYP1A2 dependent metabolism of caffeine in man. *Br. J. Clin. Pharmacol.*, **35**(4), 431–6.

Gelernter, J. , Kranzler, H. *et al.* (1997). Serotonin transporter protein (SLC6A4) allele and haplotype frequencies and linkage disequilibria in African- and European-American and Japanese populations and in alcohol-dependent subjects. *Hum. Genet.*, **101**(2), 243–6.

Goldstein, J. A. , Ishizaki, T. *et al.* (1997). Frequencies of the defective CYP2C19 alleles responsible for the mephenytoin poor metabolizer phenotype in various Oriental, Caucasian, Saudi Arabian and American black populations. *Pharmacogenetics*, **7**(1), 59–64.

Greenberg, B. D. , McMahon, F. J. *et al.* (1998). Serotonin transporter candidate gene studies in affective disorders and personality: promises and potential pitfalls. *Mol. Psychiatry*, **3**(3), 186–9.

Hariri, A. R. & Weinberger, D. R. (2003). Functional neuroimaging of genetic variation in serotonergic neurotransmission. *Genes Brain Behav.*, **2**(6), 341–9.

Jurima-Romet, M. , Crawford, K. *et al.* (1994). Terfenadine metabolism in human liver. In vitro inhibition by macrolide antibiotics and azole antifungals. *Drug Metab. Dispos.*, **22**(6), 849–57.

Kelly, C. & McCreadie, R. G. (1999). Smoking habits, current symptoms, and premorbid characteristics of schizophrenic patients in Nithsdale, Scotland. *Am. J. Psychiatry*, **156**(11), 1751–7.

Kim, H. , Lim, S. W. *et al.* (2006). Monoamine transporter gene polymorphisms and antidepressant response in Koreans with late-life depression. *JAMA*, **296**(13), 1609–18.

Le Marchand, L. , Sivaraman, L. *et al.* (1998). Associations of CYP1A1, GSTM1, and CYP2E1 polymorphisms with lung cancer suggest cell type specificities to tobacco carcinogens. *Cancer Res.*, **58**(21), 4858–63.

Leathart, J. B. , London, S. J. , *et al.* (1998). CYP2D6 phenotype-genotype relationships in African-Americans and Caucasians in Los Angeles. *Pharmacogenetics*, **8**(6), 529–41.

Lin, K., Elwyn, T. S. , *et al.* (2004). *Culture and Drug Therapy in Clinician's Guide to Cultural Psychiatry*. Amsterdam: Elsevier.

Lin, K. M. & Cheung, F. (1999). Mental health issues for Asian Americans. *Psychiatr. Serv.,* **50**(6), 774–80.

Lin, K. M. & Poland, R. E. (1995). *Ethnicity, Culture, and Psychopharmacology in Psychopharmacology: The Fourth Generation of Progress.* New York; NY: Raven Press.

Lin, K. M. , Poland, R. E. *et al.* (1988). Haloperidol and prolactin concentrations in Asians and Caucasians. *J. Clin. Psychopharmacol.,* **8**(3), 195–201.

Lin, K. M. , Poland, R. E. *et al.* (1989). A longitudinal assessment of haloperidol doses and serum concentrations in Asian and Caucasian schizophrenic patients. *Am. J. Psychiatry,* **146**(10), 1307–11.

Lin, K. M., Poland, R. E. *et al.* (1993). *Psychopharmacology and Psychobiology of Ethnicity.* Washington, DC: American Psychiatric Press.

Lin, K. M. & Smith, M. W. (2000). *Psychopharmacotherapy in the Context of Culture and Ethnicity. Ethnicity and Psychopharmacology.* Washington, DC: American Psychiatric Association.

Lin, K. M., Smith, M. W. *et al.* (2003). *Psychopharmacology: Ethnic and Cultural Perspectives.* Psychiatry. Chichester: John Wiley & Sons.

Liou, Y. H., Lin, C. T. *et al.* (2006). The high prevalence of the poor and ultrarapid metabolite alleles of CYP2D6, CYP2C9, CYP2C19, CYP3A4, and CYP3A5 in Taiwanese population. *J. Hum. Genet.,* **51**(10), 857–63.

Lohr, J. B. & Flynn, K. (1992). Smoking and schizophrenia. *Schizophr. Res.,* **8**(2), 93–102.

Masimirembwa, C. M. & Hasler, J. A. (1997). Genetic polymorphism of drug metabolising enzymes in African populations: implications for the use of neuroleptics and antidepressants. *Brain. Res. Bull.,* **44**(5), 561–71.

Mendoza, R. , Wan, Y. J. *et al.* (2001). CYP2D6 polymorphism in a Mexican American population. *Clin. Pharmacol. Ther.,* **70**(6), 552–60.

Miller, L. G. (1989). Recent developments in the study of the effects of cigarette smoking on clinical pharmacokinetics and clinical pharmacodynamics. *Clin. Pharmacokinet.,* **17**(2), 90–108.

Ng, J., Lin, K. M. *et al.* (2005). *Perspectives in Cross-Cultural Psychiatry.* Philadelphia, PA: Lippincott Williams & Wilkins.

Oesterheld, J. & Kallepalli, B. R. (1997). Grapefruit juice and clomipramine: shifting metabolitic ratios. *J. Clin. Psychopharmacol.,* **17**(1), 62–3.

Pollock, B. G. , Ferrell, R. E. *et al.* (2000). Allelic variation in the serotonin transporter promoter affects onset of paroxetine treatment response in late-life depression. *Neuropsychopharmacology,* **23**(5), 587–90.

Rausch, J. L. , Johnson, M. E. *et al.* (2002). Initial conditions of serotonin transporter kinetics and genotype: influence on SSRI treatment trial outcome. *Biol. Psychiatry,* **51**(9), 723–32.

Roby, C. A. , Anderson, G. D. *et al.* (2000). St John's Wort: effect on CYP3A4 activity. *Clin. Pharmacol. Ther.,* **67**(5), 451–7.

Roh, H. K. , Dahl, M. L. *et al.* (1996). Debrisoquine and S-mephenytoin hydroxylation phenotypes and genotypes in a Korean population. *Pharmacogenetics,* **6**(5), 441–7.

Schein, J. R. (1995). Cigarette smoking and clinically significant drug interactions. *Ann. Pharmacother.,* **29**(11), 1139–48.

Schildkraut, J. J. , Kopin, I. J. *et al.* (1995). Norepinephrine metabolism and psychoactive drugs in the endogenous depressions. 1968. *Pharmacopsychiatry,* **28** (1): 24–37.

Smeraldi, E. , Zanardi, R. *et al.* (1998). Polymorphism within the promoter of the serotonin transporter gene and antidepressant efficacy of fluvoxamine. *Mol. Psychiatry,* **3**(6), 508–11.

Wang, S. L. , Huang, J. D. *et al.* (1993). Molecular basis of genetic variation in debrisoquin hydroxylation in Chinese subjects: polymorphism in RFLP and DNA sequence of CYP2D6. *Clin. Pharmacol. Ther.,* **53**(4), 410–18.

Xie, H. G. , Stein, C. M. *et al.* (1999). Allelic, genotypic and phenotypic distributions of S-mephenytoin 4′-hydroxylase (CYP2C19) in healthy Caucasian populations of European descent throughout the world. *Pharmacogenetics,* **9**(5), 539–49.

Yoshida, K. , Ito, K. *et al.* (2002). Influence of the serotonin transporter gene-linked polymorphic region on the antidepressant response to fluvoxamine in Japanese depressed patients. *Prog. Neuropsychopharmacol. Biol. Psychiatry,* **26**(2), 383–6.

Yu, Y. W. , Tsai, S. J. *et al.* (2002). Association study of the serotonin transporter promoter polymorphism and symptomatology and antidepressant response in major depressive disorders. *Mol. Psychiatry,* **7**(10), 1115–19.

Zanardi, R. , Serretti, A. *et al.* (2001). Factors affecting fluvoxamine antidepressant activity: influence of pindolol and 5-HTTLPR in delusional and nondelusional depression. *Biol. Psychiatry,* **50**(5), 323–30.

Zevin, S. & Benowitz, N. L. (1999). Drug interactions with tobacco smoking. An update. *Clin. Pharmacokinet.,* **36**(6), 425–38.

# 4

# Ethnic differences in psychotropic drug response and pharmacokinetics

Timothy Lambert and Trevor R. Norman

## Introduction

There is increasing awareness that ethnic and cultural influences can alter individual responses to medications (Lambert & Minas, 1998). Ethno-psychopharmacology investigates cultural variations and differences that influence the effectiveness of prescription medicines used in the treatment of mental illnesses. Differences in response can be explained by both genetic and psychosocial variations. They range from genetic variants in drug metabolism to cultural practices, which may affect diet, adherence to prescribed patterns of medication use, placebo response, and the simultaneous use of traditional and alternative healing methods (Lin *et al.*, 1991).

However, predictions regarding genetic expression based on ethnicity alone need to be exercised with caution. Although connections between ethnicity and drug metabolism were recognized early, for example primaquine induced hemolysis based on G6PD deficiency in some Afro-Americans (Alving *et al.*, 1956), such differences are based more on genetic endowment per se rather than racial or ethnic divisions. The validity of therapy based solely on racial differences has been questioned, for example, in relation to differential drug responses in cardiology for Black and White patients (Schwartz, 2001).

All populations irrespective of racial group exhibit substantial intra-population variability (Jorde & Wooding, 2004). Within a single racial population between 93 and 95% of all human genetic variability is captured (Jones & Perlis, 2006). A small amount of genetic variation ($\sim$0.02% of all nucleotides) distinguishes populations from each other and no single marker can identify race or ancestry. On the other hand, self-reported race has been shown to correlate with genetic variation (Sinha *et al.*, 2006). Thus, while specific knowledge of both the genotypic and phenotypic profile may be necessary to accurately predict individual metabolic

*Ethno-psychopharmacology: Advances in Current Practice*, eds. C. H. Ng, K.-M. Lin, B. S. Singh and E. Y. K. Chiu. Published by Cambridge University Press. © C. H. Ng, K.-M. Lin, B. S. Singh and E. Y. K. Chiu 2008.

function, ethnicity remains a useful and important clinical consideration in pharmacotherapy. Nevertheless other variables, such as age, gender, hepatic/ renal function, weight, and physical status, also need to be considered in tailoring individual dosage of medication. Awareness of ethno-psychopharmacological principles is expected to improve treatment effectiveness for different ethnic groups.

### Genetic factors influencing drug response

There are wide ethnic variations in drug metabolism due to genetic variations in the drug-metabolizing enzymes. For the most part genetic variations are responsible for reductions in the activity of a number of drug-metabolizing enzymes resulting in higher amounts of medication in the blood potentially resulting in untoward side effects. For example, 33% of African Americans and 37% of Asians are slow metabolizers of several antipsychotic and antidepressant medications (Lin, Anderson & Poland 1997). Awareness of such factors should lead to more cautious prescribing practices, which entail patients starting at lower doses in the beginning of treatment. In clinical practice the opposite is often true. For example more oral doses and injections of antipsychotic drugs are often prescribed in African American patients than Caucasians in psychiatric emergency services (Segal, Bola & Watson, 1996), a clinical finding that may not be warranted from the pharmacokinetic and pharmacodynamic data to hand (Lawson, 1996; Jeste *et al.*, 1996). Slow metabolism combined with overmedication of antipsychotic drugs in African Americans can yield excessive extrapyramidal side effects (Lin *et al.*, 1997). These are the kinds of experiences that likely contribute to the mistrust of mental health services reported among African Americans (Sussman, Robins & Eavis, 1987).

### Non-genetic factors influencing drug responses: dietary and sociocultural

Among non-genetic factors contributing to the activity of liver enzymes are diet, nicotine, alcohol, caffeine, drugs, and other substances. Induction of the enzyme CYP3A4 has been observed with concomitant use of the herbal treatment of depression, St. John's Wort (*Hypericum perforatum*). Use of this herb can result in the increased metabolism of CYP3A4 substrates (Lin, Smith & Ortiz, 2001). Similarly, substances found in foods such as charbroiled beef, cruciferous vegetables (cabbage and sprouts), high-protein diet (Anderson *et al.*, 1991) and constituents of tobacco (DeVane, 1994) can induce the enzyme CYP1A2. Inhibition of certain hepatic CYP enzymes has been noted with concurrent use of grapefruit juice, which contains narigenin (Fuhr, 1998) an inhibitor of CYP3A4, the enzyme responsible for metabolism of a number of psychotropic medications. Common food ingredients may inhibit CYP1A2 for example flavinoids, quercetin (from corn), and some ingredients of coffee. Some Chinese herbs are substrates for drug-metabolizing enzymes and may potentially interact with CYP enzymes although this has not been studied systematically (Lin *et al.*, 2001). Sociocultural considerations represent another dimension affecting pharmacotherapeutic response. Cross-cultural issues regarding diagnosis, beliefs, and expectations about treatment and its outcome, compliance with prescribed medication, placebo effect, and use of traditional treatments may all impact on drug responses in more potent ways than biological mechanisms (Lin & Smith, 2000). These cultural factors can influence perceptions held about psychiatric drugs. As such the implicit attitudes of patients have been correlated with treatment adherence to medications. Negative perceptions about psychotropic medications are frequently associated with non-compliance and poor therapeutic response (Awad *et al.*, 1995). Expectation exerts an important role in the clinical effects of pharmacotherapy. Generally at least a third of subjects in most antidepressant drug trials experience a placebo response (Swartzman & Burkell, 1998). The underlying mechanism for this effect is not well understood and has been largely attributed to non-specific factors in therapy such as the nature of the doctor–patient relationship that occurs during treatment. Transcultural studies suggest that patients from non-Western cultures are likely to present with somatic symptoms of psychiatric disorders. This could be related to the absence of a mind–body dualism in non-Western medical systems where symptoms are often regarded as a disharmony in an integrated entity (Ng, 1997). Consequently, some somatic symptoms may be attributed to the side effects of medication and be perceived as intolerance to Western drugs. This in turn may lead to premature discontinuation of psychotropic drugs or to non-compliance. Thus culturally related attitudes and expectations affect both the placebo response rate and the experience of adverse reactions to pharmacotherapy.

## Pharmacogenetic differences in drug metabolism

It is well recognized that there are marked inter-individual differences in response to the same medication. The difference between individuals tends to be larger than that between the same person measured at different times (or between monozygotic twins) (Vesell, 1989). It has been estimated that up to 90% of the observed variance in drug disposition and response is due to genetic variance (Kalow, Tang & Endrenyi, 1998). For example it has been noted that drug plasma concentrations can vary more than 600-fold between individuals of the same weight and height for the same dose of drug (Eichelbaum, Ingelman-Sundberg & Evans, 2006). Although non-genetic factors such as age, organ function, diet, and drug interactions also influence the effects of medication, there are numerous examples of the genetic influence on both pharmacokinetic and pharmacodynamic responses to medications (Evans & Relling, 1999; Ng *et al.*, 2004; Evans & Johnson, 2001).

## Drug-metabolizing enzymes

The most important enzymes, and by far the most extensively studied group, for drug metabolism are the cytochrome P450 (CYP) group (Nelson, 1999). At least 17 gene families have been identified in mammals (Lin & Lu, 2001). These enzyme families can be divided into two main classes: those involved with the synthesis of bio-steroids, fatty acids, and bile acids and those involved primarily with the metabolism of xenobiotics. The majority of drug metabolism is accomplished by three main families of enzyme: CYP1, CYP2, and CYP3. The liver contains an abundance of these enzymes and is well recognized as the primary source of drug metabolism. Drug-metabolizing enzymes are also present in other tissues such as the mucosa of the intestine, kidney, lung, brain, and skin (Krishna & Klotz, 1994). Among these sites the mucosa of the intestine is probably the most important for extra-hepatic metabolism of drugs. Characteristically CYP enzymes show wide inter-individual and inter-ethnic variations in expression of the enzyme protein. For example, Shimada *et al.* (1994) studied the enzyme content from 30 Caucasian and 30 Japanese donors. For individual enzyme subtypes, differences in content were approximately 5-fold for CYP2C and CYP3A4, 12-fold for CYP2E1, 20-fold for CYP1A2, and >50-fold for CYP2A6, CYP2B6, and CYP2D6. Similar variability has been reported by other investigators (Paine *et al.*, 1997; Thummel *et al.*, 1994). As catalytic activity is higher for a given substrate due to the higher enzyme content, large variability can be expected for both hepatic and intestinal metabolism of drugs.

Genetic variation in drug-metabolizing enzymes results in different metabolic levels of functioning classified into four metabolic phenotypic groups: normal or extensive metabolizers (EMs) with normal to high metabolic activity; poor metabolizers (PMs) with low to absent metabolic activity; intermediate metabolizers (IMs) with impaired or slow metabolic function, the efficiency lying somewhere between PMs and EMs; and ultra-rapid metabolizers (UMs) with extreme metabolic activity stemming from functional gene duplication/multiplication, leading to rapid metabolism and excretion of drugs (Lin *et al.*, 2001; Pi & Gray, 1998). Differences in the metabolic clearance rates of substrates between these groups may result for example in different toxicity risks from medications. Furthermore there may be under-dosing of medication in some patients leading to reduced efficacy or therapeutic failure.

The various metabolic phenotypes are associated with variants in the gene(s) coding for the particular drug-metabolizing enzyme. Mutant alleles may differ from normal functioning (or "wild type") alleles by a single-point mutation, gene deletions, or gene duplications. The production of alternate forms of the same drug-metabolizing enzyme by gene mutations results in the varieties of phenotypic expression noted above (Meyer, 2000). Thus EMs are homozygous for active alleles; IMs are homozygous or heterozygous for partial active alleles; PMs are homozygous for defective alleles; and UMs have duplicate or multiple copies of the active gene(s) (Kirchheiner *et al.*, 2001).

Over 70 variant alleles have been identified for CYP2D6, but only a few mutations are common accounting for >95% of polymorphisms (Meyer, 2000). The *CYP2D6\*1* and *CYP2D6\*2* are active alleles, while *CYP2D6\*9*, *CYP2D6\*10*, and *CYP2D6\*17*, are partially active alleles. Major alleles responsible for deficits in enzyme activity include *CYP2D6\*3*, *CYP2D6\*4*, *CYP2D6\*5*, *CYP2D6\*6*, and *CYP2D6\*7*, while *CYP2D6\*8*, *CYP2D6\*14*, and *CYP2D6\*16* are rare deficient alleles (Daly *et al.*, 1996). For the isoenzyme CYP2C19, the active allele is *CYP2C19\*1* while the main deficient alleles are *CYP2C19\*2* and *CYP2C19\*3*. Extensive metabolizer phenotypes are either homozygous or heterozygous genotypes for the active allele, while PMs have homozygous deficient genotypes (Poolsup, Li & Knight, 2000). The isoenzyme CYP2C19 does not appear to be associated with any UM variants (Daniel & Edeki, 1996). At least three variants of the enzyme CYP2C9, which constitutes about 20% of total hepatic P450 content, have been identified (Inoue *et al.*, 1997). The wild type, designated *CYP2C9\*1*, and two mutants *CYP2C9\*2*, *CYP2C9\*3* have been found to differ with respect to the intrinsic clearance (Vmax/Km) of different substrates (Miners *et al.*, 2000). The *CYP2C9\*2* variant is associated with impaired metabolism of S-warfarin, for example (Rettie *et al.*, 1994). The CYP3A subfamily is the predominant P450 isoenzyme in human liver (~30% of total content), of which CYP3A4 is important for the metabolism of about 50% of commonly prescribed medications (Guengerich, 1999). At least four allelic variants of the gene for CYP3A4 have been identified (Xie *et al.*, 2001). The common variant is *CYP3A4\*1B*, which results in a modest reduction of activity but probably does not significantly alter metabolism of CYP3A4 drugs (Ball *et al.*, 1999). A second allelic variant, *CYP3A4\*2*, is relatively uncommon and may alter kinetics in a substrate dependent manner (Sata *et al.*, 2000).

While genetic polymorphisms have been identified for CYP1A2 and other CYP isoenzymes, data on their functional activity is limited.

The effect of multiple active gene copies of a particular enzyme has been demonstrated in subjects with multiple copies of the *CYP2D6\*2* gene and the 10-hydroxylation of nortriptyline (Dalen *et al.*, 1998). Single oral doses of the drug were administered to subjects with 0, 1, 2, 3, and 13 functional copies of the gene and the pharmacokinetics determined. Apparent oral clearance of nortriptyline increased proportionately with the number of gene copies. The amount of the 10-hydroxy-nortriptyline metabolite formed, on the other hand, increased in proportion to the number of gene copies. Genotyping may be of practical benefit in individual patients to detect a-priori rapid clearance of a therapeutic substance.

The uridine diphosphate-glucuronosyltransferases (UGTs) family plays a major role in the excretion of endobiotics and xenobiotics and their metabolites, producing products that are more water soluble, less toxic, and more readily excreted than the parent compounds (De Leon, 2003). There are two major families of these enzymes. A number of psychotropic agents are metabolized by these enzymes including tricyclic antidepressants (TCAs), some antipsychotics (e.g., clozapine, olanzapine), some benzodiazepines (e.g., lorazepam), and mood stabilizers. Human UGT1A4 catalyzes the glucuronidation of primary, secondary, and tertiary amines, androgens, and progestins. Polymorphisms in this enzyme group may also explain some intra- and inter-ethnic variation in psychotropic metabolism (Mori *et al.*, 2005). In general, the phase II UGT metabolic aspects of psychotropics have received less attention than the phase I CYP-based metabolic pathways. Therefore ethnic variations are yet to be described in detail.

### Ethnic differences in medication metabolism

The oxidative metabolism of antipsychotics, antidepressants, and anxiolytic medications are predominantly metabolized by cytochrome P450 isoenzymes (CYP), especially CYP2D6, CYP2C19, CYP1A2, and CYP3A4. The functioning of these enzymes exhibits distinct differences across ethnic groups (Lin *et al.*, 1996). Within ethnic groups there are also significant intra-group variations resulting in differences between individuals. Metabolism, among the various component parts of pharmacokinetics, is regarded as the most significant factor in determining inter-individual and inter-ethnic differences.

Psychotropic drug responses vary between different ethnic groups. Thus it has been shown that Asian patients are likely to respond to lower doses of some psychotropics and are more likely to experience side effects. Such differences have been related to genetic polymorphisms of enzymes affecting drug metabolism, particularly the isoenzymes CYP2D6 and CYP2C19 (Pi & Gray, 1998; Lin *et al.*, 1996). Compared to the 3–6% of Caucasians who are poor metabolizers of CYP2C19, 15–30% of Asians are PMs while 2–4% of Africans are PMs. Prevalent within Asian populations are the deficient genotypes, *CYP2C19\*2* and *CYP2C19\*3*, which are predictive of PM phenotypes with low metabolic activity (Goldstein *et al.*, 1997; Roh *et al.*, 1996). With respect to the other major psychotropic drug-metabolizing isozyme CYP2D6, about 5–10% of Caucasians and 1–2% of Asians are PMs (Poolsup *et al.*, 2000). On the other hand the mutant allele, *CYP2D6\*10* an intermediate functioning allele, is carried by up to 50% of Asians. A high incidence of IMs with impaired metabolic capacity is likely in Asian populations (Lin *et al.*, 1996). Inter-ethnic differences in CYP3A4-mediated drug metabolism have been studied using Caucasian and Japanese liver microsomes (Shimada *et al.*, 1994). The activity of Caucasian liver microsomes toward nifedipine oxidation and testosterone

6ß-hydroxylation was significantly higher than for Japanese. Together with other studies on different substrates the data suggest that CYP3A4 activity is higher in Caucasians than Asian populations (Xie *et al.*, 2001). This is supported by single-dose ethno-pharmacokinetic data for benzodiazepines metabolized by CYP3A4 (see below). The common variant is *CYP3A4*1B* with markedly different distributions for ethnic populations: 3.6–11% in White and Hispanic subjects, absent in Chinese and Japanese while in Black populations there is a high frequency (53–69%). A second allelic variant designated *CYP3A4*2* is low in White populations (2.7%) and was not observed in Black or Chinese groups (Xie *et al.*, 2001; Tayeb *et al.*, 2000). Both of these variants appear to contribute only modestly to changes in drug metabolism, and their clinical relevance is yet to be firmly determined.

## Antidepressant ethnic differences

### Pharmacokinetic differences

Asian subjects have an increased likelihood of carrying genetic polymorphisms that result in significantly lower metabolic clearance rates for drugs that are substrates for CYP enzymes. There are consequent clinical implications for pharmacotherapy in these subjects. At standard doses serum drug concentrations may be higher with an ensuing higher incidence of side effects and increased sensitivity to both short- and long-term adverse effects (Gray & Pi, 1998). Lower tolerance to medication would result in poor compliance rates while there may also be an increased risk of drug–drug interactions and toxicity during multiple drug treatment. Thus, lower medication doses are frequently prescribed for optimal therapeutic benefit in Asian patients (Gray & Pi, 1998; Meyer *et al.*, 1996). Differential polymorphism rates between ethnic groups have implications for drug development where the clinical drug-trial findings in one group (usually Caucasians) are frequently extrapolated to another group without qualification.

Studies of differences in the pharmacokinetics of individual antidepressant agents between ethnic groups have been conducted since the mid 1970s (see Table 4.1 for a summary of some of these studies). The majority of these studies were performed without knowledge of the polymorphisms of the liver enzymes discussed above. Interpretation of the findings based on ethnicity per se is therefore limited. Much of the difference observed is, in all probability, accounted for by the different distribution of various genotypes within the particular ethnic cohorts. This is illustrated by more recent studies examining the effect of allelic variants of particular enzymes on the pharmacokinetics of single doses of various antidepressants within a particular ethnic group. A few examples illustrate the point. The kinetics of nortriptyline and its 10-hydroxy metabolite was studied in 15 healthy Chinese volunteers (Yue *et al.*, 1998). The study showed that the *CYP2D6*10* allele was associated with higher plasma concentrations compared to those subjects with the *CYP2D6*1* allele. This

**Table 4.1** Some pharmacokinetic studies of antidepressants in different ethnic groups

| Drug and dose | Populations (N) | Results | Reference |
| --- | --- | --- | --- |
| Clomipramine (25, 50 mg) | Caucasian (11) Indian/Pakistani (6) | Cmax higher Indian/Pakistani | Allen *et al.*, 1977 |
| Desipramine (100 mg) | Caucasian (16) Chinese (14) | Cmax DMI, OH-DMI higher in Chinese | Rudorfer *et al.*, 1984 |
| Nortriptyline (100 mg) | Caucasian (10) Japanese (10) | Cmax, Tmax not different | Kishimoto & Hollister, 1984 |
| Desipramine (50, 75 mg) | Caucasian (20) Asian (20) | Tmax shorter Asians | Pi *et al.*, 1986 |
| Nortriptyline (75 mg) | Hispanic (10) Caucasian (10) | No differences | Gaviria *et al.*, 1986 |
| Desipramine (1 mg/kg) | Caucasian (19) Asian (18) | Tmax shorter in Caucasians | Pi *et al.*, 1989 |
| Sertraline (50 mg/day) | Caucasian (15) Chinese (Australia) (17) Chinese (Malaysia) (13) | No differences steady state sertraline | Ng *et al.*, 2006a |

was due to an impaired conversion of nortriptyline to 10-hydroxy-nortriptyline. Since the frequency of this allele is as high as 50% in Chinese subjects and relatively rare (<5%) in Caucasians, differences in kinetics for nortriptyline (and other CYP2D6 substrates) are explained by the presence (or absence) of the allele per se not necessarily by ethnicity. Similar data are observed for the single dose kinetics of venlafaxine in Japanese subjects, who along with Chinese and Koreans, have similar frequencies of the *CYP2D6\*10* allele (Fukuda *et al.*, 2000). Subjects with the defective alleles *CYP2C19\*2* and *CYP2C19\*3* also showed higher concentrations of venlafaxine than those without the alleles. These particular alleles are also implicated in the metabolism of amitriptyline in Japanese subjects (Shimoda *et al.*, 2002).

## Pharmacodynamic differences

Genetic factors affect pharmacodynamic responses to medication as well as determining the pharmacokinetics of drugs. The pharmacogenetic approach has been applied to the prediction of responses to drugs based on genetic subtypes of drug receptors, transporters, or other targets believed to be important for therapeutic outcome. This burgeoning field and its application to psychopharmacotherapeutics have been described in detail elsewhere (Serretti, Lilli & Smeraldi, 2002; Malhotra, Murphy & Kennedy, 2004; Lee, 2005; Binder & Holsboer, 2006). It is beyond the scope of this chapter to provide more than an illustration applicable to the response to antidepressants. A prime target of action of selective serotonin re-uptake inhibitors (SSRIs) is the serotonin transporter protein. Several polymorphisms have been described for the gene controlling this protein (Lesch *et al.*, 1993). In particular the insertion/deletion of a 44 base pair region produces a short (S) and long (L) allele. Although the serotonin transporter gene linked polymorphic region (5HTTLPR) was described as bi-allelic there are some rare (<5%) very long and extra long alleles described in Japanese and African American populations (Gelernter *et al.*, 1999). Numerous variants also occur within the repeat of this gene. The long allele leads to higher serotonin re-uptake by the transporter protein. More than 20 studies have examined the relationship between polymorphisms in this gene and response to antidepressant, mostly SSRI, treatment (these are described in detail in the following chapter on pharmacogenetics). In Caucasian patients there is an association between the long allele and better clinical response to SSRIs compared to those depressed patients with the short allelic variant (Yu *et al.*, 2002; Smeraldi *et al.*, 1998; Zanardi *et al.*, 2000; Pollock *et al.*, 2000; Zanardi *et al.*, 2001). In Asian patients the finding is not entirely consistent as results in Korean, Japanese, and Chinese depressed subjects suggest an association between the S-allele and clinical response (Kim *et al.*, 2000; Yoshida *et al.*, 2002; Ito *et al.*, 2002; Ng, Norman, Ho *et al.*, 2006b). Such discrepancies may be accounted for by ethnic differences in the transporter gene but have not been adequately studied.

Associations between antidepressant drug response and several other gene candidates have been investigated. Replicated positive associations for G-protein β 3-subunit and tryptophan hydroxylase type 1 (TPH1) have been published and reviewed (Binder & Holsboer, 2006). For these genes there is a suggestion that ethnic differences may also influence the outcome of such studies. Thus an association of an intronic single nucleotide polymorphism (SNP) in TPH1 with response to fluvoxamine and paroxetine was replicated in Caucasian samples but not a Japanese cohort (Yoshida *et al.*, 2002). Such association studies are at an early stage of development and the influence of ethnic differences has not been fully researched.

## Benzodiazepine ethnic differences

The isozyme CYP3A4 is responsible for the clearance of a number of benzodiazepine anxiolytics and hypnotics (Rendic & Di Carlo, 1997). As noted above, there are significant inter-ethnic differences in various alleles for this enzyme, which may result in significantly different pharmacokinetics for substrates of this enzyme. Thus alprazolam oral and systemic clearance was lower in Asians than in Caucasians, but similar in American born and native Asians (Lin *et al.*, 1988a). On the other hand, the pharmacokinetics of the two short-acting hypnotic agents, midazolam and triazolam, were comparable between ethnic groups (Wandel *et al.*, 2000; Kinirons *et al.*, 1996). The apparent oral clearance and bioavailability of midazolam was similar in African and Caucasian American men (Wandel *et al.*, 2000). Oral clearance of triazolam was similar for Asian Indians and Caucasians (Kinirons *et al.*, 1996).

These differences may become particularly germane if co-prescribing with some antipsychotics is undertaken. For example, in certain individuals, combinations of clozapine with benzodiazepines may lead to unexpected adverse events, including delirium and augmented respiratory depression (Jackson, Markowitz & Brewerton, 1995; Grohmann *et al.*, 1989). Presumably if there are additive or synergistic effects of ethnicity on clearance of one or both substances, adverse events may be enhanced. Similar interactions are theoretically possible with olanzapine, as adverse interactions have been described between olanzapine and benzodiazepines, at least in the elderly (Kryzhanovskaya *et al.*, 2006).

## Antipsychotic ethnic differences

Ethno-psychopharmacological studies of antipsychotics are sparse, often contradictory, and have been asserted to be methodologically flawed (Poolsup *et al.*, 2000). Problems with studies to date include poorly defined samples with imprecise definitions of various ethnic groups ("Asians" may include somewhat disparate groups such as Vietnamese, Japanese, Malaysian, Chinese, etc.), underpowered sample sizes, poor study design often using convenience samples, variable use of diagnostic criteria, lack of control of factors known to influence pharmacokinetics (such as diet, age, gender, weight, smoking), and the lack of examination of pharmacodynamic differences (Pi, 1998).

### Pharmacokinetic differences

It is clear that ethnic differences in response to antipsychotics exist (Emsley *et al.*, 2002; Frackiewicz *et al.*, 1997). Whereas there has been some work examining first-generation antipsychotics (FGAs) (for reviews, see Frackiewicz *et al.*, 1997; Poolsup *et al.*, 2000), there remains a considerable dearth of research that has examined ethnic differences with respect to the second-generation antipsychotics (SGAs).

One approach to formulating potential differences in ethnic response is to examine the metabolic pathways of the common antipsychotics and determine whether the known ethnic variations in metabolizing enzymes or other effects on absorption, distribution, and excretion can be applied a priori to predict potential clinical effects. In this section we will consider some of the commonly prescribed SGAs, and only briefly touch on the FGAs.

### First-generation antipsychotics

The findings with FGAs suggest that compared to Caucasians, Asians require lower doses, higher plasma levels, or lower neuroleptic thresholds (Collazo *et al.*, 1996;

Chiu *et al.*, 1992; Lin & Finder, 1983; Lin *et al.*, 1988b; Potkin *et al.*, 1984; Lin *et al.*, 1989; Ruiz *et al.*, 1996; Jann *et al.*, 1989; Jann *et al.*, 1992; Zhang-Wong *et al.*, 1998). The majority of these studies were carried out with haloperidol. A number of studies examined differences between Caucasians and Hispanics, and African Americans and Caucasians (Midha *et al.*, 1988b; Midha *et al.*, 1988a; Ruiz *et al.*, 1996). In general these studies provided mixed results. Another noteworthy feature of the research literature is that there appear to be no studies that have considered ethnic differences in pharmacokinetics and response for the depot antipsychotics. This may be an artifact of the low levels of depot prescribing found in the US, China, and Japan.

However, taken as a whole, the findings from these early studies did point the way to considering ethnicity as an important variable in psychopharmacological response to antipsychotics. It is unfortunate that despite the rapid increase in the development of SGAs, and the voluminous literature accompanying them, specific clinical studies of the influence of ethnicity remain uncommon.

### Second-generation antipsychotics

The main metabolic pathways and psychotropic agents that may be co-prescribed and act as inducers/inhibitors are shown in Table 4.2.

### Clozapine

Clozapine is principally metabolized by CYP1A2 followed by 2C19, 3A4, 2C9, and 2D6. Whereas clinically CYP1A2 and 2C19 are considered the key oxidative isoforms and 2C9 and 2D6 play a relatively minor role, 3A4 may play a more substantial role in the presence of high clozapine concentrations (Olesen & Linnet, 2001). As noted elsewhere, differences between ethnic groups when considering CYP3A4 metabolism may more reflect the effect of environmental factors than any genetic polymorphisms. For substrates of this CYP2C19 isozyme, variability in the efficiency of the EMs is found, depending on whether there exists a homozygous or heterozygous wild type allele, and this may be helpful in explaining both inter-individual and ethnic differences. Asians have higher frequencies of the heterozygous active allele than Caucasians (Poolsup *et al.*, 2000).

CYP1A2 is the major isozyme for clozapine oxidative metabolism, accounting for 70% of clozapine's metabolism (Bertilsson *et al.*, 1994). 1A2 does not exhibit any clinically meaningful polymorphisms in the active enzyme but polymorphisms do exist in the region of the genome that may confer differing sensitivity to the effect of inducers (Murray, 2006). This may account for some ethnic variations depending on exposure to environmental inducing agents, such as smoking (Todesco *et al.*, 2003). However, in general, genetic variations probably explain less than 1% of patients requiring very high or very low doses of clozapine (de Leon, Armstrong & Cozza, 2005b). However, individuals may carry differing quantities of CYP1A2, and

**Table 4.2** Principal enzymes involved in metabolism of second-generation antipsychotics

| SGAs "atypical" antipsychotics | Metabolism | Inducers | Inhibitors |
|---|---|---|---|
| Risperidone Aripiprazole | 2D6 > 3A4 2D6, 3A4 | Carbamazepine and phenytoin; topiramate; hypericum (St. John's Wort). | Paroxetine, fluoxetine, sertraline (high dose); grapefruit juice; 2D6 or 3A4 substrates acting as competitive inhibitors. |
| Olanzapine Clozapine | 1A2 > UGT1A4; FMO3 1A2 ≫ 2C19>3A4> 2C9>2D6; UGT1A4; FMO3 | Smoking; lamotrigine; broccoli and charbroiled food. | Fluvoxamine; fluoxetine; sertraline (high dose); caffeine; CYP1A2 substrates (TCAs). |
| Quetiapine | 3A4 ≫ 2D6, 2C9 | Carbamazepine and phenytoin; topiramate; prednisolone. | Fluvoxamine; fluoxetine; sertraline (high dose); CYP3A4 substrates; grapefruit juice. |
| Ziprasidone | Cytosolic aldehyde-oxidase; 3A4 | | |
| Amisulpride | Direct excretion | | |

SGAs = second-generation antipsychotics (SGAs); FMO3 = flavin-containing monooxygenase;
TCAs = tricyclic antidepressants
Adapted from de Leon *et al.*, 2005b

in general females have lower 1A2 activity compared to males, and gender effects may be accentuated during pregnancy.

The effects of smoking are probably more powerful moderators than any genetic variants in CYP1A2. In particular the gender by smoking interaction should alert clinicians to possible differences in effectiveness. That different ethnic groups have different smoking habits and that gender-based smoking differences exist, suggests that clozapine and olanzapine variations may be a function of these two variables (Kaholokula *et al.*, 2006). Further, caffeine, a common constituent of many diets, is an inhibitor of CYP1A2. Thus those with higher caffeine intakes have higher clozapine blood levels and lower norclozapine/clozapine ratios (Raaska, Raitasuo, Laitila *et al.*, 2004).

Beyond phase I metabolism, clozapine is a substrate for UTT1A4 and polymorphisms have already been identified in Japanese populations (Mori *et al.*, 2005). Presumably other populations will display some variability. How this relates to everyday clinical practice is as yet unknown.

In terms of the clinical use of clozapine, clear ethnic differences in dosing have been identified. Compared to the higher doses required by Caucasians, Asian patients require lower doses to achieve an effective plasma concentration (Ng et al., 2005; Chang et al., 1997; Matsuda et al., 1996). Ng et al. (2005) found that even after controlling for body weight, cigarette smoking, and caffeine intake, Asian patients had a significantly higher plasma clozapine/dose ratio than a matched Caucasian group.

With respect to other ethnic groups, African Americans may have a differential sensitivity to weight gain on clozapine (de Leon et al., 2007). They may also require lower doses than Caucasians (Kelly et al., 2006) and inter-individual as well as ethnic responsiveness may be partly explained by differences in dopamine receptor polymorphisms (Hwang et al., 2005). It is conceivable that side effects may also be differentially expressed based on pharmacodynamic differences resulting from polymorphisms in other receptor types (histaminergic, muscarinic, etc.). This area remains largely unexplored with respect to ethnic differences in antipsychotic side effects.

## Olanzapine

As might be expected from its structure, olanzapine shares many metabolic similarities to clozapine. In terms of oxidative metabolism CYP1A2 produces N-desmethyl-olanzapine and 7-OH olanzapine (perhaps accounting for 50–60% of olanzapine's metabolism [de Leon et al., 2005b]), CYP2D6 catalyzes 2-OH olanzapine formation and flavin-containing monooxygenase (FMO3) is responsible N-oxide olanzapine formation (Ring et al., 1996). Whereas there appears to be ethnic diversity in FMO3 genotypes, at this point in time the role of such variations remains a potential target for understanding differences in abnormal metabolism or adverse drug reactions (Cashman et al., 2001). However, the role of phase II UGT1A4 metabolism may be more important in olanzapine than CYP1A2 is to clozapine as direct conjugation forms a major part of olanzapine's metabolism (Caccia, 2000; Linnet, 2002). As noted above, ethnic variations in UGT1A4 and their relationship to ethnic variations in olanzapine (and clozapine) disposition are yet to be widely studied.

Smoking plays a similar but diminished role in reducing olanzapine levels as it does for clozapine (Botts, Littrell & Leon, 2004). Given the different rates of smoking in different ethnic groups, it has been suggested that caffeine phenotyping may be useful in setting an individual's olanzapine dose; clozapine may also be a candidate for routine testing (Carrillo et al., 2003).

There is little published information that directly examines ethnic differences in olanzapine pharmacokinetics or pharmacodynamics. Indirectly, examining stable prescribing patterns may indicate real-world, clinician-adjusted doses that account for factors including ethnicity (Liu *et al.*, 2003). To date, olanzapine doses appear to be only marginally lower in Asians than Caucasians and it is uncertain whether this is to do with confounders such as smoking, age, or gender (Weiss *et al.*, 2005). Side effects will require further examination. The issue of increased sensitivity to the development of type 2 diabetes in many Asian populations would warrant particular attention in situations where antipsychotics cause particular weight gain (Lee *et al.*, 2006; Ananth *et al.*, 2005).

### Risperidone

Risperidone is a very commonly prescribed SGA, in both the Western and in Asian countries. Risperidone is metabolized by CYP2D6 primarily and to a lesser extent, CYP3A4 (Wu & McKown, 2000). As discussed above, the gene encoding the CYP2D6 enzyme is highly polymorphic and the variants are distributed unequally among ethnic populations. Asians have a large proportion carrying the less efficient alleles, particularly 2D6 *10 (Japanese 40%, Koreans 50%, Chinese up to 70%) (Xie *et al.*, 2001), resulting in "slow" or "intermediate" metabolizers. This is in keeping with the finding that many Asian patients require lower doses of risperidone than their Caucasian counterparts (Luo *et al.*, 2004). Those of African descent are more likely to carry the *17 allele, another partially active allele. This has been estimated to have only one-fifth of the metabolic capacity of the wild-type allele. There appears to be some evidence that PMs of risperidone do have significantly more adverse drug reactions and, importantly, much higher risks of discontinuing the drug (de Leon *et al.*, 2005a).

The result of having reduced capacity CYP2D6 enzymes is that the antipsychotic and side effect threshold doses are lowered. Reports of Asian doses are often less than for Caucasians, but not in all cases (Zhou *et al.*, 2006; Lane *et al.*, 2001; Lee *et al.*, 2006). It is unfortunate that most studies do not report on the CYP2D6 genotypes of their study patients, which most likely accounts for the wide variability. In keeping with the general principle that Asian patients should start with low doses is the further confounder of episode status. In general first-episode patients, usually more sensitive than multi-episode patients, would be expected to have even lower doses. Available evidence suggests that this is the case, for example in studies of predominantly Chinese patients (mean risperidone dose $1.47 \pm 0.56$ mg/day) (Verma *et al.*, 2005).

### Aripiprazole

Aripiprazole shares a similar metabolic profile to risperidone, being metabolized by CYP2D6 and 3A4 (Kubo *et al.*, 2005). Few studies exist to compare and contrast aripiprazole effects in different ethnic groups. A recent study indicated that Chinese patients responded very similarly to Caucasian patients on a fixed dose of 15 mg/day (Chan *et al.*, 2007). At doses between 10 and 30 mg/day there is little incremental change in the apparent occupancy of D2 receptors (Yokoi *et al.*, 2002). Aripiprazole's partial dopaminergic agonism appears to obviate EPS in this dose range, and this wide therapeutic index may "mask" the adverse effects of high plasma levels that occur with poor 2D6 metabolizers (in contrast to the situation seen with risperidone poor metabolizers [de Leon *et al.*, 2005a]). Considering aripiprazole's complex pharmacology, pharmacodynamic studies examining well defined ethnic cohorts would be revealing. The reputation for being more metabolically neutral than other SGAs also requires specific examination, especially given the increased sensitivity of non-Caucasian populations to the development of type 2 diabetes (Carulli *et al.*, 2005).

## Ziprasidone

Ziprasidone is mainly metabolized by cytosolic aldehyde oxidase, with 3A4 playing a minor role (de Leon *et al.*, 2005b; Beedham, Miceli & Obach, 2003). Cytosolic aldehyde oxidase does not appear to demonstrate any genetic polymorphisms and this suggests that doses are likely to be similar across ethnic groups. Like quetiapine, the minor 3A4 component of ziprasidone's metabolism may be responsive to changes in environment. However, it appears as though ziprasidone is only marginally affected by 3A4 inducers such as carbamazepine (Miceli *et al.*, 2000). Thus any differences arising across ethnic groups would not be expected based on phase I oxidative metabolism. As noted for aripiprazole, future studies of ziprasidone in populations sensitive to the development of diabetes should examine this agent's reputation for reduced weight gain, and thus, decreased diabetogenic potential.

## Quetiapine

Quetiapine is predominantly metabolized by CYP3A4. Environmental rather than genetic differences are most likely to explain unusual differences in the serum concentration to dose ratio for this antipsychotic (de Leon *et al.*, 2005b).

## Amisulpride

As amisulpride has no hepatic metabolism, low protein binding, and is directly excreted in urine, there is little reason to suspect pharmacokinetic ethnic differences. Of course body mass and pharmacodynamic differences might occur, but to date have received little investigative attention.

## Drug–drug interactions

As noted above, very many patients are treated with poly-psychotropic pharmacy. For the majority of those receiving antipsychotics (patients with schizophrenia and bipolar disorder), co-therapy with other psychotropics is high (Janssen *et al.*, 2004; Sim *et al.*, 2004). This is of importance to considering inter-ethnic differences as the type and degree of polypharmacy in different settings may affect the metabolism, and ultimately the apparent dosing and effectiveness of antipsychotics.

In some Asian studies fluvoxamine has been purposely used as a means of raising clozapine doses through its role in inhibiting CYP1A2 (Lu *et al.*, 2000). This practice requires careful monitoring of plasma clozapine levels. One interesting effect derived from such studies is the finding that fluvoxamine-augmented clozapine treatment results in a lower nor-clozapine level with the suggestion of a relative decrease in metabolic consequences (Lu *et al.*, 2004).

As can be seen in Table 4.2, many agents commonly co-prescribed with antipsychotics may act as inducers and inhibitors. That these agents are also prone to ethnically determined variations in their own metabolism, suggests that providing the optimal dose of antipsychotics in various ethnic groups may become complex where psychotropic polypharmacy is common.

### Pharmacodynamic differences

Although earlier work with FGAs suggested pharmacodynamic differences across ethnic groups (Lin *et al.*, 1988b), comparative ethnic pharmacodynamic studies relating to antipsychotic effectiveness of the SGAs appear to be in their infancy. As noted above, polymorphisms in the dopamine receptor gene have been postulated to account for pharmacodynamic differences in response to antipsychotics such as clozapine and risperidone (Hwang *et al.*, 2005; Xing *et al.*, 2006a). Further details are described in the following chapter. Whereas a broad range of candidate genes may bear fruit including the serotonin transporter (Wang *et al.*, 2007) and the P-glycoprotein producing gene ABCB1 (Xing *et al.*, 2006b), it is likely that as the science of pharmacogenomics expands, an increasing number of potential genetic mechanisms may be identified that may help further in our understanding of ethnic responses to antipsychotics.

### Conclusion

Ethnic differences have been shown to influence response to psychotropic medications. Much of the focus on the explanation for such differences has been on drug-metabolizing (CYP) enzymes of the liver and their sway over pharmacokinetic factors. It is now well recognized that differences in the distribution of polymorphic variants of CYP enzymes exist between different ethnic groups. However, within ethnic groups there are considerable inter-individual variations in drug kinetics, which may not be accounted for solely by genetic variation. Responses to pharmacotherapy are multifaceted and involve the interaction of environmental and cultural factors in addition to genetic ones. In particular environmental factors may play a significant role in altering pharmacokinetics, but are often inadequately considered (Lin & Smith, 2000). For example, consumption of drugs or chemicals that are potent enzyme inhibitors may convert an EM phenotype to a PM phenotype. Dietary factors, herbal medication, chemicals, and environmental pollutants are exogenous agents that have been shown to alter the activity of drug-metabolizing enzymes, particularly CYP1A2 and CYP3A4 (Lin & Smith, 2000). Dietary habits are socioculturally determined but their influence on drug metabolism remains poorly understood for the most part. Asians and Africans exposed to a Western diet and environment do not necessarily exhibit the same sensitivity to psychotropics as those living in their native countries (Allen, Rack & Vaddadi, 1977). Variations in diet and lifestyle common to a given ethnic group have the potential to determine differences in drug response.

The application of pharmacogenetic principles to psychotropic drug response has the potential to improve outcomes for patients but must not be considered in isolation. Expression of polymorphic genes controlling brain function and drug-metabolizing enzymes are also influenced by epigenetic factors. Response to treatment can be affected by culture, attitudes to medication, and prescribing practices. The complex interplay between these factors in different ethnic groups and clinical settings requires further research. Despite the advances in gene technology and its ever-growing application to the problem of pharmacotherapy, there remains a need to strive for "holistic" evaluation of the individual patient and practice the "art" of medicine to ensure optimal care (Ng *et al.*, 2004).

## REFERENCES

Allen, J. J., Rack, P. H. & Vaddadi, K. S. (1977). Differences in the effects of clomipramine on English and Asian volunteers. Preliminary report on a pilot study. *Postgrad. Med. J.*, **53**(4), 79–86.

Alving, A. S. *et al.* (1956). Enzymatic deficiency in primaquine-sensitive erythrocytes. *Science*, **124**, 484–5.

Ananth, J. *et al.* (2005). Atypical antipsychotic drugs, diabetes and ethnicity. *Expert Opin. Drug Saf.*, **4**, 1111–24.

Anderson, K. E. *et al.* (1991). Diet and cimetidine induce comparable changes in theophylline metabolism in normal subjects. *Hepatology*, **13**, 941–6.

Awad, A. G. *et al.* (1995). Patients' subjective experiences on antipsychotic medications: implications for outcome and quality of life. *Int. Clin. Psychopharmacol.*, **10**(3), 123–32.

Ball, S. E. *et al.* (1999). Population distribution and effects on drug metabolism of a genetic variant in the 5′ promoter region of CYP3A4. *Clin. Pharmacol. Ther.*, **66**, 288–94.

Beedham, C., Miceli, J. J. & Obach, R. S. (2003). Ziprasidone metabolism, aldehyde oxidase, and clinical implications. *J. Clin. Psychopharmacol.*, **23**, 229–32.

Bertilsson, L. *et al.* (1994). Clozapine disposition covaries with CYP1A2 activity determined by a caffeine test. *Br. J. Clin. Pharmacol.*, **38**, 471–3.

Binder, E. B. & Holsboer, F. (2006). Pharmacogenomics and antidepressant drugs. *Ann. Med.*, **38**, 82–94.

Botts, S., Littrell, R. & de Leon, J. (2004). Variables associated with high olanzapine dosing in a state hospital. *J. Clin. Psychiatry*, **65**, 1138–43.

Caccia, S. (2000). Biotransformation of post-clozapine antipsychotics: pharmacological implications. *Clin. Pharmacokinet.*, **38**, 393–414.

Carrillo, J. A. *et al.* (2003). Role of the smoking-induced cytochrome P450 (CYP)1A2 and polymorphic CYP2D6 in steady-state concentration of olanzapine. *J. Clin. Psychopharmacol.*, **23**, 119–27.

Carulli, L. *et al.* (2005). Review article: diabetes, genetics and ethnicity. *Aliment. Pharmacol. Ther.*, **22**(2), 16–19.

Cashman, J. R. *et al.* (2001). Population distribution of human flavin-containing monooxygenase form 3: gene polymorphisms. *Drug Metab. Dispos.*, **29**, 1629–37.

Chan, H. Y. *et al.* (2007). Efficacy and safety of aripiprazole in the acute treatment of schizophrenia in Chinese patients with risperidone as an active control: a randomized trial. *J. Clin. Psychiatry*, **68**, 29–36.

Chang, W. H. *et al.* (1997). Clozapine dosages and plasma drug concentrations. *J. Formos. Med. Assoc.*, **96**, 599–605.

Chiu, H. *et al.* (1992). Neuroleptic prescription for Chinese schizophrenics in Hong Kong. *Aust. N. Z. J. Psychiatry*, **26**, 262–4.

Collazo, Y. *et al.* (1996). Neuroleptic dosing in Hispanic and Asian Inpatients with schizophrenia. *Mt. Sinai. J. Med.*, **63**, 310–13.

Dalen, P. *et al.* (1998). 10-Hydroxylation of nortriptyline in white persons with 0, 1, 2, 3, and 13 functional CYP2D6 genes. *Clin. Pharmacol. Ther.*, **63**, 444–52.

Daly, A. K. *et al.* (1996). Nomenclature for human CYP2D6 alleles. *Pharmacogenetics*, **6**, 193–201.

Daniel, H. I. & Edeki, T. I. (1996). Genetic polymorphism of S-mephenytoin 4′-hydroxylation. *Psychopharmacol. Bull.*, **32**, 219–30.

de Leon, J. (2003). Glucuronidation enzymes, genes and psychiatry. *Int. J. Neuropsychopharmacol.*, **6**, 57–72.

de Leon, J. *et al.* (2005a). The CYP2D6 poor metabolizer phenotype may be associated with risperidone adverse drug reactions and discontinuation. *J. Clin. Psychiatry*, **66**, 15–27.

de Leon, J., Armstrong, S. C. & Cozza, K. L. (2005b). The dosing of atypical antipsychotics. *Psychosomatics*, **46**, 262–73.

de Leon, J. *et al.* (2007). Weight gain during a double-blind multidosage clozapine study. *J. Clin. Psychopharmacol.*, **27**, 22–7.

DeVane, C. L. (1994). Pharmacogenetics and drug metabolism of newer antidepressant agents. *J. Clin. Psychiatry*, **55**(38–45) 46–7.

Eichelbaum, M., Ingelman-Sundberg, M. & Evans, W. E. (2006). Pharmacogenomics and individualized drug therapy. *Annu. Rev. Med.*, **57**, 119–37.

Emsley, R. A. *et al.* (2002). Ethnicity and treatment response in schizophrenia: a comparison of 3 ethnic groups. *J. Clin. Psychiatry*, **63**, 9–14.

Evans, W. E. & Johnson, J. A. (2001). Pharmacogenomics: the inherited basis for interindividual differences in drug response. *Annu. Rev. Genomics Hum. Genet.*, **2**, 9–39.

Evans, W. E. & Relling, M. V. (1999). Pharmacogenomics: translating functional genomics into rational therapeutics. *Science*, **286**, 487–91.

Frackiewicz, E. J. *et al.* (1997). Ethnicity and antipsychotic response. *Ann. Pharmacother.*, **31**, 1360–9.

Fuhr, U. (1998). Drug interactions with grapefruit juice. Extent, probable mechanism and clinical relevance. *Drug Saf.*, **18**, 251–72.

Fukuda, T. *et al.* (2000). The impact of the CYP2D6 and CYP2C19 genotypes on venlafaxine pharmacokinetics in a Japanese population. *Eur. J. Clin. Pharmacol.*, **56**, 175–80.

Gaviria, M., Gil, A. A. & Javaid J. I. (1986). Nortriptyline kinetics in Hispanic and Anglo subjects. *J. Clin. Psychopharmacol.*, **6**, 227–31.

Gelernter, J. *et al.* (1999). Population studies of polymorphisms of the serotonin transporter protein gene. *Am. J. Med. Genet.*, **88**, 61–6.

Goldstein, J. A. *et al.* (1997). Frequencies of the defective CYP2C19 alleles responsible for the mephenytoin poor metabolizer phenotype in various Oriental, Caucasian, Saudi Arabian and American black populations. *Pharmacogenetics*, **7**, 59–64.

Gray, G. E. & Pi, E. H. (1998). Ethnicity and medication-induced movement disorders. *J. Pract. Psychiatry Behav. Health*, **5**, 259–64.

Grohmann, R. *et al.* (1989). Adverse effects of clozapine. *Psychopharmacology*, **99**, S101–4.

Guengerich, F. P. (1999). Cytochrome P-450 3A4: regulation and role in drug metabolism. *Annu. Rev. Pharmacol. Toxicol.*, **39**, 1–17.

Hwang, R. *et al.* (2005). Association study of 12 polymorphisms spanning the dopamine D(2) receptor gene and clozapine treatment response in two treatment refractory/intolerant populations. *Psychopharmacology*, **181**, 179–87.

Inoue, K. *et al.* (1997). Relationship between CYP2C9 and 2C19 genotypes and tolbutamide methyl hydroxylation and S-mephenytoin 4′-hydroxylation activities in livers of Japanese and Caucasian populations. *Pharmacogenetics*, **7**, 103–13.

Ito, K. *et al.* (2002). A variable number of tandem repeats in the serotonin transporter gene does not affect the antidepressant response to fluvoxamine. *Psychiatry Res*, **111**, 235–9.

Jackson, C. W., Markowitz, J. S. & Brewerton, T. D. (1995). Delirium associated with clozapine and benzodiazepine combinations. *Ann. Clin. Psychiatry*, **7**, 139–41.

Jann, M. W. *et al.* (1989). Haloperidol and reduced haloperidol plasma levels in Chinese vs. non-Chinese psychiatric patients. *Psychiatry Res.*, **30**, 45–52.

Jann, M. W. *et al.* (1992). Comparison of haloperidol and reduced haloperidol plasma levels in four different ethnic populations. *Prog. Neuropsychopharmacol. Biol. Psychiatry*, **16**, 193–202.

Janssen, B. *et al.* (2004). Validation of polypharmacy process measures in inpatient schizophrenia care. *Schizophr. Bull.*, **30**, 1023–33.

Jeste, D. V. *et al.* (1996). Relationship of ethnicity and gender to schizophrenia and pharmacology of neuroleptics. *Psychopharmacol. Bull.*, **32**, 243–51.

Jones, D. S. & Perlis, R. H. (2006). Pharmacogenetics, race, and psychiatry: prospects and challenges. *Harv. Rev. Psychiatry*, **14**, 92–108.

Jorde, L. B. & Wooding, S. P. (2004). Genetic variation, classification and 'race'. *Nat. Genet.*, **36**, S28–33.

Kaholokula, J. K. *et al.* (2006). Ethnic-by-gender differences in cigarette smoking among Asian and Pacific Islanders. *Nicotine Tob. Res.*, **8**, 275–86.

Kalow, W., Tang, B. K. & Endrenyi, L. (1998). Hypothesis: comparisons of inter- and intra-individual variations can substitute for twin studies in drug research. *Pharmacogenetics*, **8**, 283–9.

Kelly, D. L. *et al.* (2006). Clozapine utilization and outcomes by race in a public mental health system: 1994–2000. *J. Clin. Psychiatry*, **67**, 1404–11.

Kim, D. K. *et al.* (2000). Serotonin transporter gene polymorphism and antidepressant response. *Neuroreport*, **11**, 215–19.

Kinirons, M. T. *et al.* (1996). Triazolam pharmacokinetics and pharmacodynamics in Caucasians and Southern Asians: ethnicity and CYP3A activity. *Br. J. Clin. Pharmacol.*, **41**, 69–72.

Kirchheiner, J. *et al.* (2001). CYP2D6 and CYP2C19 genotype-based dose recommendations for antidepressants: a first step towards subpopulation-specific dosages. *Acta Psychiatr. Scand.*, **104**, 173–92.

Kishimoto, A. & Hollister, L. (1984). Nortriptyline kinetics in Japanese and Americans. *J. Clin. Psychopharmacol.*, **4**, 171–2.

Krishna, D. R. & Klotz, U. (1994). Extrahepatic metabolism of drugs in humans. *Clin. Pharmacokinet.*, **26**, 144–60.

Kryzhanovskaya, L. A. *et al.* (2006). A review of treatment-emergent adverse events during olanzapine clinical trials in elderly patients with dementia. *J. Clin. Psychiatry*, **67**, 933–45.

Kubo, M. *et al.* (2005). Influence of itraconazole co-administration and CYP2D6 genotype on the pharmacokinetics of the new antipsychotic Aripriprazole. *Drug Metab. Pharmacokinet.*, **20**, 55–64.

Lambert, T. J. R. & Minas, I. H. (1998). Transcultural psychopharmacology and pharmacotherapy. *Australasian Psychiatry*, **6**, 61–4.

Lane, H. Y. *et al.* (2001). A pilot double-blind, dose-comparison study of risperidone in drug-naive, first-episode schizophrenia. *J. Clin. Psychiatry*, **62**, 994–5.

Lawson, W. B. (1996). Clinical issues in the pharmacotherapy of African-Americans. *Psychopharmacol. Bull.*, **32**, 275–81.

Lee, C. *et al.* (2006). Treatment with olanzapine, risperidone or typical antipsychotic drugs in Asian patients with schizophrenia. *Aust. N. Z. J. Psychiatry*, **40**, 437–45.

Lee, M. S. (2005). The pharmacogenetics of antidepressant treatments for depressive disorders. *Drug Dev. Res.*, **65**, 170–8.

Lesch, K. P. *et al.* (1993). Isolation of a cDNA encoding the human brain serotonin transporter. *J. Neural Transm. Gen. Sect.*, **91**, 67–72.

Lin, J. H. & Lu, A. Y. (2001). Interindividual variability in inhibition and induction of cytochrome P450 enzymes. *Annu. Rev. Pharmacol. Toxicol.*, **41**, 535–67.

Lin, K. M. & Finder, E. (1983). Neuroleptic dosage for Asians. *Am. J. Psychiatry*, **140**, 490–1.

Lin, K. M. & Smith, M. W. (2000). Psychopharmacotherapy in the context of culture and ethnicity. In P. Ruiz, ed., *Ethnicity and Psychopharmacology*. Washington, DC: American Psychiatric Press, pp. 1–36.

Lin, K. M. *et al.* (1988a). Comparison of alprazolam plasma levels in normal Asian and Caucasian male volunteers. *Psychopharmacology*, **96**, 365–9.

Lin, K. M. *et al.* (1988b). Haloperidol and prolactin concentrations in Asians and Caucasians. *J. Clin. Psychopharmacol.*, **8**, 195–201.

Lin, K. M. *et al.* (1989). A longitudinal assessment of haloperidol doses and serum concentrations in Asian and Caucasian schizophrenic patients. *Am. J. Psychiatry*, **146**, 1307–11.

Lin, K. M. *et al.* (1991). Pharmacokinetic and other related factors affecting psychotropic responses in Asians. *Psychopharmacol. Bull.*, **27**, 427–39.

Lin, K. M. *et al.* (1996). The evolving science of pharmacogenetics: clinical and ethnic perspectives. *Psychopharmacol. Bull.*, **32**, 205–17.

Lin, K. M., Anderson, D. & Poland, R. E. (1997). Ethnic and cultural considerations in psychopharmacotherapy. In D. Dunner, ed., *Current Psychiatric Therapy II*. Philadelphia, PA: WB Saunders, pp. 75–81.

Lin, K. M., Smith, M. W. & Ortiz, V. (2001). Culture and psychopharmacology. *Psychiatr. Clin. North Am.*, **24**, 523–38.

Linnet, K. (2002). Glucuronidation of olanzapine by cDNA-expressed human UDP-glucuronosyltransferases and human liver microsomes. *Hum. Psychopharmacol.*, **17**, 233–8.

Liu, C. Y. *et al.* (2003). Optimal dose of risperidone and olanzapine for patients with schizophrenia in Taiwan. *Int. Clin. Psychopharmacol.*, **18**, 49–51.

Lu, M. L. *et al.* (2000). Fluvoxamine reduces the clozapine dosage needed in refractory schizophrenic patients. *J. Clin. Psychiatry*, **61**, 594–9.

Lu, M. L. *et al.* (2004). Adjunctive fluvoxamine inhibits clozapine-related weight gain and metabolic disturbances. *J. Clin. Psychiatry*, **65**, 766–71.

Luo, N. *et al.* (2004). Drug utilization review of risperidone for outpatients in a tertiary referral hospital in Singapore. *Hum. Psychopharmacol.*, **19**, 259–64.

Malhotra, A. K., Murphy, G. M. J. & Kennedy, J. L. (2004). Pharmacogenetics of psychotropic drug response. *Am. J. Psychiatry*, **161**, 780–96.

Matsuda, K. T. *et al.* (1996). Clozapine dosage, serum levels, efficacy, and side-effect profiles: a comparison of Korean-American and Caucasian patients. *Psychopharmacol. Bull.*, **32**, 253–7.

Meyer, U. A. (2000). Pharmacogenetics and adverse drug reactions. *Lancet*, **356**, 1667–71.

Meyer, U. A. *et al.* (1996). Antidepressants and drug-metabolizing enzymes – expert group report. *Acta Psychiatr. Scand.*, **93**, 71–9.

Miceli, J. J. *et al.* (2000). The effect of carbamazepine on the steady-state pharmacokinetics of ziprasidone in healthy volunteers. *Br. J. Clin. Pharmacol.*, **49**(1), 65S–70S.

Midha, K. K. *et al.* (1988a). Variation in the single dose pharmacokinetics of fluphenazine in psychiatric patients. *Psychopharmacology*, **96**, 206–11.

Midha, K. K. *et al.* (1988b). A pharmacokinetic study of trifluoperazine in two ethnic populations. *Psychopharmacology*, **95**, 333–8.

Miners, J. O. *et al.* (2000). Torsemide metabolism by CYP2C9 variants and other human CYP2C subfamily enzymes. *Pharmacogenetics*, **10**, 267–70.

Mori, A. *et al.* (2005). UDP-glucuronosyltransferase 1A4 polymorphisms in a Japanese population and kinetics of clozapine glucuronidation. *Drug Metab. Dispos.*, **33**, 672–5.

Murray, M. (2006). Role of CYP pharmacogenetics and drug–drug interactions in the efficacy and safety of atypical and other antipsychotic agents. *J. Pharm. Pharmacol.*, **58**, 871–85.

Nelson, D. R. (1999). Cytochrome P450 and the individuality of species. *Arch. Biochem. Biophys.*, **369**, 1–10.

Ng, C. H. (1997). The stigma of mental illness in Asian cultures. *Aust. N. Z. J. Psychiatry*, **31**, 382–90.

Ng, C. H. *et al.* (2004). The emerging role of pharmacogenetics: implications for clinical psychiatry. *Aust. N. Z. J. Psychiatry*, **38**, 483–9.

Ng, C. H. *et al.* (2005). An inter-ethnic comparison study of clozapine dosage, clinical response and plasma levels. *Int. Clin. Psychopharmacol.*, **20**, 163–8.

Ng, C. H., Norman, T. R., Ho, B. *et al.* (2006a). A comparison study of sertraline dosages, plasma levels, efficacy and adverse reactions in Chinese versus Caucasian populations. *Int. Clin. Psychopharmacol.*, **21**, 87–92.

Ng, C. H., Easteal, S., Tan, S. *et al.* (2006b). Serotonin transporter polymorphisms and clinical response to sertraline across ethnicities. *Progress in Neuropsychopharmacology and Biological Psychiatry*, **30**, 953–7.

Olesen, O. V. & Linnet, K. (2001). Contributions of five human cytochrome P450 isoforms to the N-demethylation of clozapine in vitro at low and high concentrations. *J. Clin. Pharmacol.*, **41**, 823–32.

Paine, M. F. *et al.* (1997). Characterization of interintestinal and intraintestinal variations in human CYP3A-dependent metabolism. *J. Pharmacol. Exp. Ther.*, **283**, 1552–62.

Pi, E. H. (1998). Transcultural psychopharmacology: present and future. *Psychiatry Clin. Neurosci.*, **52**, S185–7.

Pi, E. H. & Gray, G. E. (1998). A cross-cultural perspective on psychopharmacology. *Essential Psychopharmacology*, **2**, 233–59.

Pi, E. H., Simpson, G. H. & Cooper, T. B. (1986). Pharmacokinetics of desipramine in Caucasian and Asian volunteers. *Am. J. Psychiatry*, **143**, 1174–6.

Pi, E. H., Tran-Johnson, T. K., Walker, N. R. *et al.* (1989). Pharmacokinetics of desipramine in Asian and Caucasian volunteers. *Psychopharmacol. Bull.*, **25**, 483–7.

Pollock, B. G. *et al.* (2000). Allelic variation in the serotonin transporter promoter affects onset of paroxetine treatment response in late-life depression. *Neuropsychopharmacology*, **23**, 587–90.

Poolsup, N., Li Wan Po, A. & Knight, T. L. (2000). Pharmacogenetics and psychopharmacotherapy. *J. Clin. Pharm. Ther.*, **25**, 197–220.

Potkin, S. G. *et al.* (1984). Haloperidol concentrations elevated in Chinese patients. *Psychiatry Res.*, **12**, 167–72.

Raaska, K., Raitasuo, V., Laitila, J. & Neuvonen, P. J. (2004). Effect of caffeine-containing versus decaffeinated coffee on serum clozapine concentrations in hospitalised patients. *Pharmacol. Toxicol.*, **94**, 13–18.

Rendic, S. & Di Carlo, F. J. (1997). Human cytochrome P450 enzymes: a status report summarizing their reactions, substrates, inducers, and inhibitors. *Drug Metab. Rev.*, **29**, 413–580.

Rettie, A. E. *et al.* (1994). Impaired (S)-warfarin metabolism catalysed by the R144C allelic variant of CYP2C9. *Pharmacogenetics*, **4**, 39–42.

Ring, B. J. *et al.* (1996). Identification of the human cytochromes P450 responsible for the in vitro formation of the major oxidative metabolites of the antipsychotic agent olanzapine. *J. Pharmacol. Exp. Ther.*, **276**, 658–66.

Roh, H. K. *et al.* (1996). Debrisoquine and S-mephenytoin hydroxylation phenotypes and genotypes in a Korean population. *Pharmacogenetics*, **6**, 441–7.

Rudorfer, M. V., Lane, E. A., Chang, W. H., Zhang, M. D. & Potter, W. Z. (1984). Desipramine pharmacokinetics in Chinese and Caucasian volunteers. *Br. J. Clin. Pharmacol.*, **17**, 433–40.

Ruiz, S. *et al.* (1996). Neuroleptic dosing in Asian and Hispanic outpatients with schizophrenia. *Mt. Sinai J. Med.*, **63**, 306–9.

Sata, F. *et al.* (2000). CYP3A4 allelic variants with amino acid substitutions in exons 7 and 12: evidence for an allelic variant with altered catalytic activity. *Clin. Pharmacol. Ther.*, **67**, 48–56.

Schwartz, R. S. (2001). Racial profiling in medical research. *N. Engl. J. Med.*, **344**, 1392–3.

Segal, S. P., Bola, J. R. & Watson, M. A. (1996). Race, quality of care, and antipsychotic prescribing practices in psychiatric emergency services. *Psychiatr. Serv.*, **47**, 282–6.

Serretti, A., Lilli, R. & Smeraldi, E. (2002). Pharmacogenetics in affective disorders. *Eur. J. Pharmacol.*, **438**, 117–28.

Shimada, T. *et al.* (1994). Interindividual variations in human liver cytochrome P-450 enzymes involved in the oxidation of drugs, carcinogens and toxic chemicals: studies with liver microsomes of 30 Japanese and 30 Caucasians. *J. Pharmacol. Exp. Ther.*, **270**, 414–23.

Shimoda, K. *et al.* (2002). The impact of CYP2C19 and CYP2D6 genotypes on metabolism of amitriptyline in Japanese psychiatric patients. *J. Clin. Psychopharmacol.*, **22**, 371–8.

Sim, K. *et al.* (2004). Antipsychotic polypharmacy in patients with schizophrenia: a multicentre comparative study in East Asia. *Br. J. Clin. Pharmacol.*, **58**, 178–83.

Sinha, M. *et al.* (2006). Self-reported race and genetic admixture. *N. Engl. J. Med.*, **354**, 421–2.

Smeraldi, E. *et al.* (1998). Polymorphism within the promoter of the serotonin transporter gene and antidepressant efficacy of fluvoxamine. *Mol. Psychiatry*, **3**, 508–11.

Sussman, L. K., Robins, L. N. & Earls, F. (1987). Treatment-seeking for depression by black and white Americans. *Soc. Sci. Med.*, **24**, 187–96.

Swartzman, L. C. & Burkell, J. (1998). Expectations and the placebo effect in clinical drug trials: why we should not turn a blind eye to unblinding, and other cautionary notes. *Clin. Pharmacol. Ther.*, **64**, 1–7.

Tayeb, M. T. *et al.* (2000). CYP3A4 promoter variant in Saudi, Ghanaian and Scottish Caucasian populations. *Pharmacogenetics*, **10**, 753–6.

Thummel, K. E. *et al.* (1994). Use of midazolam as a human cytochrome P450 3A probe: II. Characterization of inter- and intraindividual hepatic CYP3A variability after liver transplantation. *J. Pharmacol. Exp. Ther.*, **271**, 557–66.

Todesco, L. *et al.* (2003). Determination of -3858G–>A and -164C–>A genetic polymorphisms of CYP1A2 in blood and saliva by rapid allelic discrimination: large difference in the prevalence of the -3858G–>A mutation between Caucasians and Asians. *Eur. J. Clin. Pharmacol.*, **59**, 343–6.

Verma, S. K. *et al.* (2005). Plasma risperidone levels and clinical response in patients with first-episode psychosis. *J. Clin. Psychopharmacol.*, **25**(6), 609–11.

Vesell, E. S. (1989). Pharmacogenetic perspectives gained from twin and family studies. *Pharmacol. Ther.*, **41**, 535–52.

Wandel, C. *et al.* (2000). CYP3A activity in African American and European American men: population differences and functional effect of the CYP3A4*1B5'-promoter region polymorphism. *Clin. Pharmacol. Ther.*, **68**, 82–91.

Wang, L. *et al.* (2007). Response of risperidone treatment may be associated with polymorphisms of HTT gene in Chinese schizophrenia patients. *Neurosci. Lett.*, **414**, 1–4.

Weiss, U. *et al.* (2005). Effects of age and sex on olanzapine plasma concentrations. *J. Clin. Psychopharmacol.*, **25**, 570–4.

Wu, W. N. & McKown, L. A. (2000). Recent advances in biotransformation of CNS and cardiovascular agents. *Curr. Drug Metab.*, **1**, 255–70.

Xie, H.-G. *et al.* (2001). Molecular basis of ethnic differences in drug disposition and response. *Annu. Rev. Pharmacol. Toxicol.*, **41**, 815–50.

Xing, Q. *et al.* (2006a). The relationship between the therapeutic response to risperidone and the dopamine D2 receptor polymorphism in Chinese schizophrenia patients. *Int. J. Neuropsychopharmacol.*, **10**, 631–7.

Xing, Q. *et al.* (2006b). Polymorphisms of the ABCB1 gene are associated with the therapeutic response to risperidone in Chinese schizophrenia patients. *Pharmacogenomics*, 7, 987–93.

Yokoi, F. *et al.* (2002). Dopamine D2 and D3 receptor occupancy in normal humans treated with the antipsychotic drug aripiprazole (OPC 14597): a study using positron emission tomography and (11C)raclopride. *Neuropsychopharmacology*, **27**, 248–59.

Yoshida, K. *et al.* (2002). Monoamine oxidase: a gene polymorphism, tryptophan hydroxylase gene polymorphism and antidepressant response to fluvoxamine in Japanese patients with major depressive disorder. *Prog. Neuropsychopharmacol. Biol. Psychiatry*, **26**, 1279–83.

Yu, Y. W. *et al.* (2002). Association study of the serotonin transporter promoter polymorphism and symptomatology and antidepressant response in major depressive disorders. *Mol. Psychiatry*, 7, 1115–19.

Yue, Q. Y. *et al.* (1998). Pharmacokinetics of nortriptyline and its 10-hydroxy metabolite in Chinese subjects of different CYP2D6 genotypes. *Clin. Pharmacol. Ther.*, **64**, 384–90.

Zanardi, R. *et al.* (2000). Efficacy of paroxetine in depression is influenced by a functional polymorphism within the promoter of the serotonin transporter gene. *J. Clin. Psychopharmacol.*, **20**(1), 105–7.

Zanardi, R. *et al.* (2001). Factors affecting fluvoxamine antidepressant activity: influence of pindolol and 5-HTTLPR in delusional and nondelusional depression. *Biol. Psychiatry*, **50**, 323–30.

Zhang-Wong, J. *et al.* (1998). An investigation of ethnic and gender differences in the pharmacodynamics of haloperidol. *Psychiatry Res.*, **81**, 333–9.

Zhou, Z. L. *et al.* (2006). Multiple dose pharmacokinetics of risperidone and 9-hydroxyrisperidone in Chinese female patients with schizophrenia. *Acta Pharmacol. Sin.*, **27**, 381–6.

# 5

# Pharmacogenetics of ethnic populations

Min-Soo Lee, Rhee-Hun Kang, and Sang-Woo Hahn

## Introduction

Highly complex mechanisms underlie the variability in drug responses, which can be attributed to several physiological and environmental factors such as age, renal and liver function, nutritional status, smoking, and alcohol consumption. However, it has been established for almost half a century that genetic factors also influence both the efficacy of a drug and the likelihood of adverse reactions (Weinshilboum, 2003). Psychotropic drugs appear to be effective across cultures and ethnicities (Lin, Poland & Nakasaki, 1993, Lin, Tsai, Yu *et al.* 1999), but it is increasingly recognized that these responses also vary (Lin & Poland, 1995; Poolsup, Li Wan Po & Knight 2000). The discovery of widespread ethnospecific polymorphisms in genes governing pharmacokinetic and pharmacodynamic aspects of psychotropic drugs may explain some of these variations (Lin *et al.*, 1999; Kalow, 1992).

## Pharmacodynamic aspects

The term pharmacodynamics encompasses all the processes that influence the relationship between drug concentration and resulting effects. Psychotropic drugs have a wide variety of targets within neurotransmitter systems, including neurotransmitter synthesis, degradation of enzymes, storage, receptors, and specific transporter proteins.

### Genetic studies of antidepressants

Serotonin transporter

The brain 5-HT transporter (5-HTT) is the principal site of action of many antidepressants. This transporter takes up 5-HT into the presynaptic neuron, thus

*Ethno-psychopharmacology: Advances in Current Practice*, eds. C. H. Ng, K.-M. Lin, B. S. Singh and E. Y. K. Chiu. Published by Cambridge University Press. © C. H. Ng, K.-M. Lin, B. S. Singh and E. Y. K. Chiu 2008.

terminating synaptic actions, and recycles it into the neurotransmitter pool. Ramamoorthy, Bauman, Moore *et al.* (1993) identified and cloned a single gene encoding the human 5-HTT, localized to chromosome 17q11.1~q12, spanning 21 kb, and consisting of 14 exons (Lesch, Balling, Gross *et al.*, 1994). A functional polymorphism (5-HTTLPR) within the promoter of the 5-HTT gene has been identified, and the in-vitro basal 5-HTT activity in carriers of the 5-HTTLPR long (l) allele was found to be more than twice that in carriers of the short (s) allele, suggesting that 5-HTT gene transcription is modulated in such variants (Ramamoorthy *et al.*, 1993; Heils, Teufel, Petri *et al.*, 1996; Lesch, Bengel, Heils *et al.*, 1996). The 5-HTTLPR s allele is reportedly associated with a poor response to selective serotonin re-uptake inhibitors (SSRIs) in Caucasian populations (Smeraldi, Zanardi, Benedetti *et al.*, 1998; Pollock, Ferrell, Mulsant *et al.*, 2000; Zanardi, Benedetti, Di Bella *et al.*, 2000; Arias, Catalan, Gasto *et al.*, 2003), and Rausch, Johnson, Fei *et al.* (2002) reported that a favorable outcome to antidepressant treatments correlated with the presence of the l allele. In contrast, Asian depressive patients (such as Koreans and Japanese) with the 5-HTTLPR s/s genotype show better responses to acute antidepressant treatments than those with other genotypes (Kim, Lim, Lee *et al.*, 2000; Yoshida, Ito, Sato *et al.*, 2002a), with the absence of the l/l genotype of intron 2 in the 5-HTT gene most powerfully predicting a non-response (Kim *et al.*, 2000). However, Yu, Tsai, Chen *et al.* (2002) reported that those with the l/l genotype had a significantly better response to SSRIs than s-allele carriers in a Chinese population. Therefore, the relationship between 5-HTTLPR genotypes and the response to antidepressant treatments remains controversial. Lee, Cha, Ham *et al.* (2004) found that 5-HTTLPR variants influence the long-term treatment outcomes of clinical improvement, responses to antidepressant treatments, age at onset, and recurrence rate after three years of antidepressant treatment. The long-term administration of serotonergic drugs is known to prevent the recurrence of depressive episodes in depression (Montgomery, 1994), which suggests that modulation of 5-HT function in the brain influences the course of mood disorders.

The genotypes of 5-HTTLPR are classified into two groups: (1) carriers of the l allele (l/l and l/s genotypes) and (2) carriers of the s/s genotype, because the l allele has been reported to have a higher 5-HTT density and activity than the s allele (Heils *et al.*, 1996; Lesch *et al.*, 1996).

The most interesting aspect of the results of the study by Lee *et al.* (2004) is that they also differ from those in a Caucasian population (Smeraldi, Benedetti & Zanardi, 2002). The authors reported a more favorable natural history in those with the s/s genotype than in l-allele carriers, which also differs from acute antidepressant responses in Caucasian populations. The frequencies of the s and l alleles among the Korean sample were approximately 86% and 14%, respectively, while the corresponding figures for Caucasians are 43% and 57% (Lesch *et al.*, 1996).

The discrepancies between the results of studies in different ethnic groups may be partially due to differences in allele frequencies.

### Tryptophan hydroxylase

Tryptophan hydroxylase (TPH) is the rate-limiting enzyme in serotonin biosynthesis. In the central nervous system, TPH is expressed in the pineal gland and brainstem raphe nuclei. The serotonergic neurons of the raphe nuclei project onto most regions of the brain, accounting for the wide range of serotonergic effects on functions such as mood, cognition, aggression, sleep, and appetite. Selective serotonin re-uptake inhibitors enhance the general serotonergic tone. Thus, the gene coding for TPH is a candidate for a possible genetic influence on the relationship between major depressive disorder (MDD) and antidepressant responses (Pickar & Rubinow, 2001). The TPH gene has been cloned (Boularand, Darmon, Ganem *et al.*, 1990) and mapped to chromosome 11p15.3-p14 (Craig, Bonlarand, Darmon *et al.*, 1991). Two biallelic polymorphisms in complete linkage disequilibrium were identified on positions 218 (A218C) and 779 (A779C) of intron 7 (Nielsen, Jenkins, Stetanisko *et al.*, 1997). Serretti *et al.* (2001a, 2001b) reported an association between the TPH A218C polymorphism and treatment responses to both fluvoxamine and paroxetine. They reported that the A/A and A/C genotypes of the TPH A218C polymorphism were associated with a worse response to paroxetine treatment, and also reported that the A/A genotype responded more slowly to fluvoxamine treatment. Ham, Lee, Lee *et al.* (2005) found no association between the TPH A218C polymorphism and antidepressant responses in 93 MDD outpatients who received various antidepressants: 41.9% received SSRIs, 26.9% received venlafaxine, 20.4% received mirtazapine, 8.6% received nefazodone, and 2.2% received tricyclic antidepressants. Yoshida, Naito, Takahashi *et al.* (2002b) also failed to demonstrate an association between TPH A218C polymorphisms and the response to fluvoxamine among Japanese patients with MDD. Whilst our study (Ham *et al.*, 2005) and that of Yoshida *et al.* (2002b) involved small samples, the discrepancy between the results of these studies and those of Serretti *et al.* (2001a, 2001b) might be due to ethnic differences.

### Serotonin receptor 2A

Serotonin receptors are other possible candidate genes involved in the pharmacogenetics of antidepressants. The concentration of 5-HTR2A receptors is high in the frontal cortex (Aroar & Melzer, 1989; Yates, Leake, Candy *et al.*, 1990). Recent experiments have shown that 5-HTR2A may mediate the antidepressant effects seen in putative animal models of anxiety and depression (Skrebuhhova, Allikmets & Matto, 1999). Moreover, positron-emission tomography has shown that antidepressant drugs decrease the density of central 5-HTR2A receptors in depressed human subjects (Yatham, Liddle & Dennie, 1999; Mayer *et al.*, 2001). The 5-HTR2A receptor is located on postsynaptic neurons and may play an important role in the effects of antidepressants (Burnet, Eastwood, Lacey *et al.*, 1995). The chronic administration of tricyclic or monoamine oxidase inhibitors results in downregulation of 5-HTR2A, and also SSRIs have been associated with a decreased responsiveness of 5-HT2 (Glennon & Dukat, 1995). Some studies have suggested that SSRIs downregulate 5-HTR2A (Maj, Bijak, Dziedzicka-Wasylewska *et al.*, 1996; Yatham *et al.*, 1999). The human 5-HTR2A gene spans 20 kb of chromosome 13 (13q14–21) (Chen, Yang, Grimsby *et al.*, 1992), and consists of three exons separated by two introns. Two common polymorphisms have been described for this gene. One polymorphism is 102T/C, which is in the non-coding region and does not alter the amino acid sequence (Erdmann, Shimron-Abarbanell, Rietschel *et al.*, 1996), but has been shown to be in absolute linkage disequilibrium with the other polymorphism, -1438A/G, that is in the promoter region (Arranz, Munro, Owen *et al.*, 1998; Spurlock, Helis, Holmas *et al.*, 1998). Cusin, Serretti, Zanardi *et al.* (2002) observed that 102T/C was marginally associated with fluvoxamine and paroxetine responses. Minov, Baghai, Schule *et al.* (2001) also investigated the relationship between 102T/C and responses to various antidepressants drugs. Choi, Kang, Ham *et al.* (2005) has also reported on the association of the -1438A/G polymorphism with antidepressant responses. The -1438G/-1438G genotype appeared to be associated with a better response to citalopram. However, our results were not consistent with those of Sato, Yoshida, Takahashi *et al.* (2002), who investigated the relationship between the -1438A/G polymorphism and the therapeutic response to fluvoxamine in 66 Japanese patients with MDD. Minov *et al.* (2001) found that a good response to antidepressant treatments was associated with the presence of the C allele of the T102C polymorphism in 5-HTR2A. Cusin *et al.* (2002) reported that the T102/T102 genotype was associated with higher HAM-D scores at baseline and poor responses to fluvoxamine and paroxetine.

### Serotonin receptor 6

The serotonin 6 (5-HT6) receptor is one of the most recently studied serotonin receptors, and an important candidate gene for the study of MDD because it is abundant in the limbic system and some antidepressants have a high affinity for it (Monsma, Shen, Ward *et al.*, 1993).

The 5-HT6 receptor is located on chromosome 1p35-p36, and the density of its mRNA is highest in the olfactory tubercle, striatum, nucleus accumbens, dentate gyrus, and cornu ammonis (CA)1, CA2, and CA3 regions of the hippocampus (Ward, Hamblin, Lachowicz *et al.*, 1995; Sleight, Boess, Bos *et al.*, 1998; Yoshioka, Matsumoto, Togashi *et al.*, 1998). 5-HT6 receptors stimulate adenylate cyclase activity via a second messenger (Kohen, Metcalf, Khan *et al.*, 1996). Several important therapeutic compounds, including tricyclic antidepressants, antipsychotics, tryptamine and ergoline derivatives, interact with the 5-HT6 receptor (Monsma *et al.*, 1993; Roth, Craigo, Choudhary *et al.*, 1994), and hence this receptor may be related to mood regulation. In humans, a silent RsaI restriction fragment length polymorphism of the 5-HT6 receptor was revealed at bp 267C/T in exon 1, corresponding to Tyr[89] (Kohen *et al.*, 1996). Vogt, Shimron-Abarbanell, Neidt *et al.* (2000) and Wu, Huo, Cheng *et al.* (2001) reported that the 5-HT6 C267T receptor polymorphism was not related to the responses to antidepressants in MDD. Lee, Lee, Lee *et al.* (2005) evaluated the association between the 5-HT6 receptor C267T polymorphism and responses of Korean patients with MDD to treatment with antidepressants. They found statistical differences in the treatment responses among three C267T genotypes after eight weeks of treatment. Patients with the CT genotype exhibited significant clinical improvements in HAM-D total, sleep, activity, and somatic anxiety scores compared with the TT genotype, but not in core, psychic anxiety, and delusion HAM-D scores.

## G-protein β3 subunit

Hundreds of cell-surface receptors for neurotransmitters and other ligands use G proteins as a messenger in intracellular signaling pathways. G proteins play important roles in determining the specificity and temporal characteristics of cellular responses to signals. Gβ proteins form dimeric complexes with Gγ subunits that interact with $G_\alpha$ subunits to generate a heterotrimeric G protein. Upon receptor activation, G proteins dissociate into free $G_\alpha$ and Gβγ subunits that can activate various effectors. Effector proteins of the Gβγ complex include phospholipases, adenylyl cyclases, ion channels, G-protein-coupled receptor kinases, and phosphoinositide-3 kinases (Ford, Skiba, Bae *et al.*, 1998; Hamm, 1998). Siffert, Rosskopf, Siffert *et al.* (1998) detected the single-nucleotide polymorphism (SNP) C825T in exon 10 of the gene encoding the β3 subunit of G protein (GNB3). The T allele of this SNP is associated with the occurrence of a splice variant (Gb3s) that leads to the deletion of 41 amino acids. The Gb3s variant has been reported to be not only associated with increased signal transduction and ion transport, but also with pathophysiological conditions such as hypertension (Benjafield, Jeyasingam, Nyholt *et al.*, 1998; Siffert *et al.*, 1998; Siffert, 2003; Dong, Zhu, Sagnella *et al.*, 1999; Hengstenberg, Schunkert, Mayer *et al.*, 2001) and obesity (Hegele, Anderson, Young *et al.*, 1999; Siffert, Forster, Jockel *et al.*, 1999). More recently, Zill, Baghai, Zwanzger *et al.* (2000) found an association between the C825T SNP of GNB3 and depression. They reported that the frequency of the T allele was significantly higher in depressive patients than in both healthy controls and schizophrenic patients. They also found a significant association between the TT genotype and responses to antidepressant treatments. Most recently, Serretti, Lorenzi, Cusin *et al.* (2003) reported the same treatment responses to SSRIs in a large sample of depressive Italian patients. Lee *et al.* (2004) tested the association between the C825T SNP and therapeutic responses to antidepressants. Major depressive disorder patients carrying the T allele have a more severe symptomatology but a better response to antidepressant treatments than patients without it.

Although this finding is consistent with previous studies in Caucasians (Bondy, Baghai, Zill *et al.*, 2002; Zill *et al.*, 2000; Siffert, 2003), it differs from a study on a Japanese population (Kunugi, Kato, Fukuda *et al.*, 2002).

According to the study by Siffert *et al.* (1999), frequencies of the T allele in Black Africans is highest (79%) while East Asians showed the intermediate values (46%) and Caucasians showed the lowest values (33%). In the Japanese sample of the study of Kunugi *et al.* (2002), the frequency of the T allele was 0.53 in both the depressive and control groups. However, in our Korean sample, the frequencies of the T allele differed significantly between the depressive and control groups, at 0.54 and 0.44, respectively. The T-allele frequency of 0.44 in our controls is similar to those in controls of Taiwanese (43.5%) (Chang, Yen, Liu *et al.*, 2002) and Chinese (47.7%) (Siffert *et al.*, 1999) populations, although it is somewhat different from another Taiwanese study (50.0%) (Lin, Tsai & Hong, 2001a).

The T allele was associated with Gb3s, the splice variant of GNB3 in which nucleotides 498–620 of exon 9 are deleted. The resulting loss of 41 amino acids produces a shortened, more-active splice variant of GNB3. There is evidence from transient-expression experiments that Gb3s is a biologically active protein that enhances signal transduction (Siffert *et al.*, 1998; Virchow, Ansorge, Rosskopf *et al.*, 1999; Rosskopf, Koch, Habich *et al.*, 2003). Rosskopf *et al.* (2003) reported that Gb3s containing G protein results in an increased number of activated Gas and free Gâγ dimers, which subsequently activate the downstream effector systems. The results of the present study suggest that the Gb3s variant related to the 825T allele is associated with vulnerability to depression and severe depressive symptoms, especially in core depressive symptoms, psychic anxiety, and delusion. Moreover, the Gb3s variant may be related to better and faster treatment responses due to enhanced signal transduction. It is interesting that the significant effects of T-allele carriers on depression and therapeutic response found in our study (Lee *et al.*, 2004) might support the dominant effect of the Gb3s variant, as has been reported previously (Siffert *et al.*, 1998). On the other hand, other studies suggest a recessive effect in the therapeutic responses of antidepressants (Zill *et al.*, 2000).

### Norepinephrine transporter

Both norepinephrine (NE) and serotonin play important roles in depression, with increased levels of NE and its metabolites commonly found in the plasma, cerebrospinal fluid, and urine of patients with MDD (Lake, Pickar, Ziegler *et al.*, 1982;

Roy, Pickar, Dejong *et al.*, 1998; Veith, Lewis, Linares *et al.*, 1994). It has been consistently reported that treating depression with selective NE-specific agents and also with serotonergic agents decreases the NE turnover (Debellis, Geracioti & Altemus, 1993; Owens, 1997). The NE transporter (NET) is responsible for the re-uptake of NE into presynaptic nerve terminals (Bonisch & Bruss, 1994). Moreover, the NET is the primary site of action for many antidepressants and secondary tricyclic amines, such as desipramine and nortriptyline (Amara & Kuhar, 1993), and desipramine treatment elevates NET mRNA in the locus coeruleus (Szot, Ashliegh, Kohen *et al.*, 1993). Likewise, the novel selective NE re-uptake inhibitor reboxetine has been observed to be at least as effective as imipramine, desipramine, and fluoxetine in the treatment of MDD (Massana, 1998; Scates, 2000). Therefore, a good candidate target for MDD treatment is the NET gene, which is located on chromosome 16q12.2, spanning approximately 45 kb and consisting of 14 exons (Porzgen, Banische & Bruss, 1995). Recently, the T → C point mutation 182 bp upstream of the first codon in the 5′-flanking promoter region of the NET gene has been identified (Zill, Engel, Baghai *et al.*, 2002). This region contains several important cis-elements for transcription (Kim, Kim, Cubells *et al.*, 1999). While the clinical and the physiological importance of NET-gene regulation is evident, the transcriptional mechanisms regulating its expression are poorly understood. Yoshida, Takahashi, Higuchi *et al.* (2004) studied how the NET genetic variants T-182C and G1287A were related to the therapeutic response to milnacipran. Ninety-six Japanese patients with MDD were treated with milnacipran at 50–100 mg/day for six weeks, and the severity of depression was assessed with the Montgomery-Asberg Depression Rating Scale. The presence of the T allele of the NET T-182C polymorphism was associated with a superior response to antidepressants, whereas the A/A genotype of the NET G1287A polymorphism was associated with a slower onset of the therapeutic response (see Table 5.1).

### Genetic studies of mood stabilizers

There have been few pharmacogenetic investigations of mood stabilizers. Selecting candidate genes for such investigations is difficult because the exact mechanisms of action of established mood stabilizers such as lithium remain uncertain (Shaldubina, Agam & Belmaker, 2001; Phiel & Klein, 2001). Serretti, Malitas, Mandelli *et al.* (2004) investigated the possible effects of genes such as COMT, MAOA, and the G-protein β3 subunit on the association between 5-HTTLPR and the efficacy of lithium. They found that subjects with the s/s variant showed a worse response to lithium. In contrast, Del Zompo, Ardua, Palmas *et al.* (1999) found no association between the efficacy of lithium and polymorphisms at the following loci: D2 receptor, D3 receptor, D4 receptor, GABA type A receptor α-1 subunit, and 5-hydroxytryptamine (5-HT)2A and 5-HT2C receptors (Serretti *et al.*, 1998,

**Table 5.1** Pharmacogenetic studies on the effects of antidepressants

| Authors | Gene | Drug | Findings | Sample | Ethnicity |
|---|---|---|---|---|---|
| Smeraldi *et al.* (1998) | SERT (5-HTTLPR) | Fluvoxamine | *l/l* and *l/s* showed a better response than *s/s*. | Major depression, bipolar depression | Caucasian |
| Pollock *et al.* (2000) | SERT (5-HTTLPR) | Paroxetine, nortriptyline | During acute treatment with paroxetine, mean reductions from baseline in HRSD were significantly more rapid for *l/l* than for *s*. The onset of the response to nortriptyline was not affected. | Late life depression | Caucasian |
| Zanardi *et al.* (2000) | SERT (5-HTTLPR) | Paroxetine | *l/l* showed a better response than *l/s* and *s/s*. | Major depression | Caucasian |
| Rausch *et al.* (2002) | SERT (5-HTTLPR) | Fluoxetine | *l* was more responsive to placebo, as well as more responsive to drug dose than was *s*. | Major depression | Caucasian |
| Arias *et al.* (2003) | SERT (5-HTTLPR) | Citalopram | *s/s* was associated with the non-remission. | Major depression | Caucasian |
| Durham *et al.* (2004) | SERT (5-HTTLPR) | Sertraline, Placebo | *l* allele showed a significant increase in response only in the sertraline group. | Major depression | Caucasian |
| Serretti *et al.* (2004) | SERT (5-HTTLPR) | Fluvoxamine, paroxetine | *s/s* variant association with a poor response. | Major depression, bipolar depression | Caucasian |
| Lee *et al.* (2004) | SERT (5-HTTLPR) | SSRIs, MAOIs, SNRIs | *ll* genotype is associated with long-term effect of antidepressant. | Major depression | Asian |
| Yoshida *et al.* (2002a) | SERT (5-HTTLPR) | Fluvoxamine | Frequency of *s* was significantly higher in responsive individuals. | Major depression | Asian |
| Kim *et al.* (2000) | SERT (5-HTTLPR) | Fluoxetine, paroxetine | *s/s* homozygosity in the promoter region showed better responses. | Major depression | Asian |

*(cont.)*

**Table 5.1** (*Cont.*)

| Authors | Gene | Drug | Findings | Sample | Ethnicity |
|---|---|---|---|---|---|
| Yu et al. (2002) | SERT (5-HTTLPR) | Fluoxetine | l/l showed significantly better responses compared with s. | Major depression | Asian |
| Cusin et al. (2002) | HTR2A (T102C) | Fluvoxamine, paroxetine | Marginal association | Major depression | Caucasian |
| Minov et al. (2001) | HTR2A (T102C) | Various antidepressants | Those with one or two C alleles of the T102C polymorphism showed significantly larger decreases. | Major depression | Caucasian |
| Murphy et al. (2003) | HTR2A (T102C) | Paroxetine, mirtazapine | Paroxetine-induced side effects were strongly associated with the HTR2A C/C genotype. | Major depression | Caucasian |
| Sato et al. (2002) | HTR2A (-1438A/G) | Fluvoxamine | No association. | Bipolar depression | Asian |
| Lee et al. (2005) | HTR2A (-1438A/G) | Citalopram | GG allele of the -1438A/G polymorphism showed better responses. | Major depression | Asian |
| Wu et al. (2001) | 5-HT6 (C267T) | Venlafaxine, fluoxetine | No association. | Major depression | Asian |
| Lee et al. (2005) | 5-HT6 (C267T) | SSRIs, SNRIs, mirtazapine nefazodone, TCAs | CT showed significantly better treatment responses than the homozygote group (CC + TT genotypes). | Major depression | Asian |
| Serretti et al. (2003) | G-protein β3 subunit (C825T) | Fluvoxamine, paroxetine | T/T variants showed better responses to treatment. | Major depression, bipolar depression | Caucasian |

| Reference | Gene (polymorphism) | Treatment | Finding | Disorder | Ethnicity |
|---|---|---|---|---|---|
| Zill et al. (2000) | G-protein β3 subunit (C825T) | TCAs, noradrenaline and specific SSRIs; SNRIs, ECT, TMS combination | TT homozygosity showed better responses to antidepressant treatments. | Major depression, bipolar depression | Caucasian |
| Lee et al. (2004) | G-protein β 3 subunit (C825T) | SSRIs, SNRIs, mirtazapine nefazodone, TCAs | T allele showed severe symptomatology but a better response. | Major depression | Asian |
| Serretti et al. (2001a) | TPH (A218C) | Paroxetine | A/A and TPH*A/C variants were associated with a poorer response to paroxetine treatment when compared to TPH*C/C. | Major depression | Caucasian |
| Serretti et al. (2001b) | TPH (A218C) | Fluvoxamine | A/A and A/C variants were associated with a worse response when compared to C/C. | Major depression, bipolar depression | Caucasian |
| Yoshida et al. (2002b) | TPH (A218C) | Fluvoxamine | No association. | Major depression | Asian |
| Lee et al. (2005) | TPH (A218C) | SSRIs, SNRIs, mirtazapine, nefazodone, TCAs | No association. | Major depression | Asian |
| Yoshida et al. (2004) | NET(T-182C) | Milnacipran | T allele of the NET T-182C polymorphism was associated with superior antidepressant responses. | Major depression | Asian |
| NET(G1287A) | | | The A/A genotype was associated with a slower onset of therapeutic response. | | |

1999, 2000). In approximately 200 bipolar and depressed patients, they found no association between lithium efficacy and polymorphisms at the loci of catechol *O*-methyltransferase, the monoamine oxidase (MAO)-A, and the G-protein β3 subunit. Moreover, in 443 bipolar and depressed patients, they found that 5-HT2A and MAO-A polymorphisms were not associated with lithium responses (Cusin *et al.*, 2002). Interpreting these results is difficult because of the diagnostic hetero-geneity of the patient groups. Furthermore, most of the candidate genes studied by these researchers were chosen for their putative association with mood disor-ders, rather than for a specific role in the mechanism of action of lithium. Bipolar disorder is considered to exhibit a high degree of heritability (Craddock & Jones, 2001), and it has been suggested that bipolar patients with a strong family history respond better to lithium (Mendlewicz, Verbancki, Linkowski *et al.*, 1978; Grof, Alda, Grof *et al.*, 1994). Turecki, Grof, Grof *et al.* (2001) performed a genome-wide search for markers linked with the lithium response in pedigrees with bipolar disease. Linkage was found between the lithium response and markers on chromo-somes 15 and 7. These interesting findings require replication in families with other characteristics.

### Genetic studies of antipsychotic drugs

Most pharmacogenetic studies into antipsychotic drugs have involved the pro-totype atypical neuroleptic clozapine. Many investigations of the influences of dopaminergic (D2, D3, and D4) receptors and serotonergic (5-HT2A, 5-HT2C, and 5-HT6) genes on the spectrum of clozapine action have produced conflicting results (see Table 5.2). Among dopamine receptors, the D3 subtype has received considerable attention due to its localization within limbic structures and its affinity to classical and atypical neuroleptics. The Ser9Gly polymorphism of the D3 receptor is associated with the action of classical neuroleptics and clozapine (Malhotra, Goldman, Buchanan *et al.*, 1998; Scharfetter, Chaudhry, Hornik *et al.*, 1999). Moreover, an association between the Ser9Gly polymorphism and the devel-opment of tardive dyskinesia has been demonstrated, suggesting that the Ser9 allele protects against the development of this disabling adverse effect (Masellis, Basile, Ozdemir *et al.*, 2000). A major candidate gene for clozapine action is the D4 recep-tor gene, since this receptor is located on the prefrontal cortex, a brain region that is thought to be linked to cognitive dysfunction in schizophrenia (Seeman & Vantol, 1994). At least two polymorphisms in the 5-HT2A receptor gene (a silent T102C exchange and a structural His452Tyr substitution) appear to play a role in the clozapine response (Basile, Masellis, Potkin *et al.*, 2002). Furthermore, a structural variant in the 5-HT2C receptor that leads to a Cys23Ser substitution might be important for responses and, more importantly, may be associated with

**Table 5.2** Pharmacogenetic studies on the effects of antipsychotic drugs

| Authors | Gene | Drug | Findings | Sample | Ethnicity |
|---|---|---|---|---|---|
| Hwu et al. (1998) | DRD4 (48-bp repeat) | Neuroleptic | Homozygous for 48-bp repeats in both is associated with good neuroleptic response during acute treatment. | Schizophrenia | Asian |
| Rao et al. (1994) | DRD4 (48-bp repeat) | Clozapine | No association. | Schizophrenia | Caucasian |
| Shaikh et al. (1995) | DRD4 (48-bp repeat) | Clozapine | No association. | Schizophrenia | Caucasian |
| Kaiser et al. (2000) | DRD4 (48-bp repeat) | Typical antipsychotic drugs, clozapine | No association. | Schizophrenia | Caucasian |
| Shaikh et al. (1996) | DRD3 (S9G) | Clozapine | s/s genotype more frequent among non-responders. | Schizophrenia | Caucasian |
| Malhotra et al. (1998) | DRD3 (S9G) | Clozapine | No association. | Schizophrenia | Caucasian |
| Scharfetter et al. (1999) | DRD3 (S9G) | Clozapine | G allele is associated with clozapine response. | Schizophrenia | Asian |
| Lin et al. (1999) | HTR2A (T102C) | Clozapine | No association. | Schizophrenia | Asian |
| Lane et al. (2002) | HTR2A (T102C) | Risperidone | C102/C102 genotype associated with a better response. | Schizophrenia | Asian |
| Joober et al. (1999) | HTR2A (T102C) | Typical antipsychotic drugs | Trend toward association between C/C genotype and poor response among men. | Schizophrenia | Caucasian |
| Arranz et al. (1998) | HTR2A (G-1438A) | Clozapine | GG genotype more common in non-responders. | Schizophrenia | Caucasian |
| | HTR2A (H452T) | Clozapine | Frequency of T allele higher in non-responders. | Schizophrenia | Caucasian |

(cont.)

**Table 5.2** (*Cont.*)

| Authors | Gene | Drug | Findings | Sample | Ethnicity |
|---|---|---|---|---|---|
| Arranz *et al.* (1996) | HTR2A (H452T) | Clozapine | T allele associated with poor response. | Schizophrenia | Caucasian |
| Arranz *et al.* (1995) | HTR2A (T102C) | Clozapine | C/C genotype associated with poor response. | Schizophrenia | Caucasian |
| Malhotra *et al.* (1996a) | HTR2A (T102C/H452T) | Clozapine, typical neuroleptics | No association. | Schizophrenia or schizoaffective disorder | Caucasian |
| Nimgaonkar *et al.* (1996) | HTR2A (T102C) | Clozapine | No association. | Schizophrenia | Caucasian |
| Nöthen *et al.* (1995) | HTR2A (T102C/H452T/ T25N) | Clozapine | No association | Schizophrenia | Caucasian |
| Malhotra *et al.* (1996b) | HTR2C (C23S) | Clozapine | No association. | Schizophrenia | Caucasian |
| Sodhi *et al.* (1995) | HTR2C (C23S) | Clozapine | S allele associated with clozapine response. | Schizophrenia | Caucasian |
| Rietschel *et al.* (1997) | HTR2C (C23S) | Clozapine | No association. | Schizophrenia | Caucasian |
| Yu *et al.* (1999) | HTR6 (C276T) | Clozapine | Homogeneous 267T/T genotype associated with better response. | Schizophrenia | Asian |
| Masellis *et al.* (2001) | HTR6 (C276T) | Clozapine | No association. | Schizophrenia | Caucasian |

**Table 5.3** Major cytochrome P isoenzymes

| Enzyme | Substrates |
| --- | --- |
| CYP1A2 | TCAs, clozapine, haloperidol, fluvoxamine, mirtazepine, olanzapine |
| CYP2D6 | TCAs, SSRIs, haloperidol, mirtazepine, zuclopenthoxil, venlafaxine, sertraline |
| CYP2C19 | TCAs, mephenytoin, diazepam, moclobemid, venlafaxine |
| CYP3A4 | TCAs, risperidone, carbamazepine, benzodiazepines, haloperidol, fluoxetine, mirtazepine, reboxetine, venlafaxine |

Adapted from Bondy & Zill, 2004

the weight gain observed with several atypical neuroleptics (Reynolds, Zhang & Zhang, 2003).

## Cytochrome P450

Drug metabolism is a critical determinant of the therapeutic and adverse effects of many psychotropic drugs. The metabolism is associated with the pharmacokinetics of a drug, which includes its absorption, distribution, and elimination. Psychotropic drugs are mainly metabolized by the cytochrome P450 (CYP) enzymes. There are approximately 20 of these enzymes, and they are often responsible for the rate-limiting step of drug metabolism. Of these, the three most commonly involved in psychotropic drug metabolism are CYP2D6, CYP3A4, and CYP2C19 (Lin, 2001b). See Table 5.3.

## CYP2D6

CYP2D6 is the best characterized P450 enzyme that exhibits polymorphism in humans. Mutations in the CYP2D6 locus can result in absent enzyme, deficient enzyme, or enzyme with increased activity (Bertilsson, 1995). Debrisoquine and sparteine, which are substrates of CYP2D6 and the first compounds shown to be subject to CYP2D6 polymorphism, are commonly used as probes when phenotyping enzyme activity (Meyer, 1994a; Gonzalez & Idle, 1994). CYP2D6 is the most extensively studied CYP isoenzyme in psychiatry. Three phenotypes have been identified so far: slow/poor metabolizers (PMs), rapid/extensive metabolizers (EMs), and ultra-rapid metabolizers (UMs) (Lin, Poland, Wan *et al.*, 1996; Meyer, 1994b). The PM trait is inherited in an autosomal recessive pattern with the gene encoding the CYP2D6 enzyme located on chromosome 22. The EMs are either homozygous for the unmutated (wild-type) gene coding for this enzyme, or heterozygous for one of the alleles with defective function. The amplification of functional CYP2D6 genes accounts for the very rapid metabolism seen in UMs. When treated with these drugs at the recommended doses, PMs often produce significantly higher plasma drug concentrations and may be more susceptible to adverse effects, whereas EMs usually show subtherapeutic plasma concentrations. The genotype of each patient prescribed these drugs is therefore potentially of great clinical significance. Altered drug metabolism may result in side effects; for example, PMs of a specific drug may metabolize that drug at a slower rate, which may prolong exposure to the drug and produce unwanted effects.

Several reports have identified associations between metabolic polymorphisms (CYP2D6*3, -*4, -*5, -*10, and CYP1A2-C/A ([first intron]) and side effects of antipsychotic therapy (tardive dyskinesia and movement disorders) (Kapitany, Meszaros, Lenzinger *et al.*, 1998; Basile, Ozdemir, Masellis *et al.*, 2000; Lam, Garcia-Barcelo, Ungvari *et al.*, 2001). The CYP2D6 and CYP2C19 subtypes participate in the metabolism of several antidepressant drugs (e.g., sertraline and fluoxetine); variants of these enzyme types that encode the PM phenotype have been associated with slower elimination rates of fluoxetine and sertraline (Hamelin, Turgeon, Vallee *et al.*, 1996; Wang, Liu, Wang *et al.*, 2001). Also, individuals with a homozygous PM genotype who receive sertraline experience adverse effects (dizziness and nausea), which may be due to toxic accumulation of the drug due to its slower elimination rate (Wang *et al.*, 2001). Thus, individual dose adjustment may be necessary for PMs to achieve the optimal therapeutic effect and avoid adverse effects (Guttendorf & Wedlund, 1992).

A notable and well established ethnicity difference in CYP2D6 expression occurs between Caucasians and Asians (Bertilsson, Lou, Du *et al.*, 1992; Lin *et al.*, 1996), with the prevalence of the PM phenotype being only 1% in Asians. Another frequently overlooked difference is that the distribution of CYP2D6 activity is significantly shifted towards lower values in Asian EMs. The molecular genetic basis of a slower CYP2D6 activity in Asian EMs was shown to result from a cytosine-to-thymine change at position (C188T) in exon 1, leading to a Pro34Ser amino acid substitution in a highly conserved region (Pro-Pro-Gly-Pro) of the CYP2D6 enzyme (Bertilsson, 1995; Johansson, Oscarson, Yue *et al.*, 1994). Importantly, this allele is highly prevalent in Asians (51% in Chinese) and causes a ten-fold decrease in catalytic activity in vivo (Johansson *et al.*, 1994). Therefore, inter-individual differences in the therapeutic and adverse effects of psychotropic drugs in Asian populations may be explained in part by the presence of the CYP2D6*10 allele. The prevalence of PMs of debrisoquine varies greatly with ethnicity, with it being highest in Caucasians and lowest in Asians. The occurrence appears to be similar in different Caucasian populations, being about 7% in Swedish Caucasians, other Europeans, and American Caucasian populations. Likewise, a comparable low prevalence of PMs, of approximately 1%, has been found in Chinese, Japanese, and Korean populations (Bertilsson *et al.*, 1992; Nakamura, Goto, Ray *et al.*, 1985; Roh, Dahl, Johansson *et al.*, 1996). The metabolic capacity for debrisoquine hydroxylation in Chinese EMs appears to be lower than that in

Caucasian EMs, but may be comparable to those in other Asian populations (Lou, 1990).

## CYP2C19

Unlike the CYP2D6 polymorphism, no UMs have been identified for the CYP2D6 polymorphic enzyme (Daniel & Edeki, 1996). The PM phenotype is inherited in an autosomal recessive fashion on chromosome 10 and occurs independently of the debrisoquine/sparteine polymorphism (Meyer, Zanger, Grant et al., 1990). The EM phenotype includes both homozygous and heterozygous genotypes for the wild-type allele(s), which is likely to be one of the reasons for the variable metabolic activities within this phenotype. Asian EMs appear to comprise more heterozygotes than homozygotes, whereas the opposite is true in Caucasians (Inaba, Nebert, Burchell et al., 1995; Kalow & Bertilsson, 1994). Only a low prevalence of PMs has been demonstrated in Caucasians (3–6%) and in African, African American, Arabic, and Caucasian populations (2–4%). By contrast, the prevalence of PMs has been shown to be 15–30% in Asian populations. Therefore, in these populations, particularly in the absence of phenotyping or genotyping, drugs metabolized by CYP2C19 should be initially prescribed at lower doses. It is noteworthy that among the substrates of CYP2C19, diazepam and omeprazole show remarkable inter-ethnic differences (Bertilsson, 1995). CYP2C19 is involved in the metabolism of several psychotropic drugs. Major ethnicity differences exist in the activity of this enzyme, from 3% to 20% for PMs. The reduced activity of this enzyme is caused by two specific mutations, one of which is specific to Asian individuals. The approximate percentage of PMs has been reported to be 20% in Asians, 5% in Hispanics, and 3% in Caucasians (de Morais, Wilkinson, Blaisdell et al., 1994; Goldstein, Ishazaki, Chiba et al., 1997). Further information on CYP nomenclature and new CYP alleles is available on the internet (http://www.imm.ki.se/CYPalleles/).

## Conclusions

Patients from different ethnic or environmental backgrounds may respond differently to psychotropic drugs, for which the underlying factors are complex. Pharmacogenetic research has uncovered significant differences among ethnic groups in the metabolism, clinical effectiveness, and side-effect profiles. The utility and possible applications of these research methodologies in the clinical setting remain to be determined. Information concerning the relative efficiency of drug-metabolizing enzymes obtained through genotyping and phenotyping methodologies could be used by clinicians who provide psychopharmacotherapeutic services to patients from diverse ethnic backgrounds (Smith & Mendoza, 1996).

## REFERENCES

Amara, S. G. & Kuhar, M. J. (1993). Neurotransmitter transporters: recent progress. *Annu. Rev. Neurosci.*, **16**, 73–93.

Arias, B., Catalan, R., Gasto, C., Gutierrez, B. & Fananas, L. (2003). 5-HTTLPR polymorphism of the serotonin transporter gene predicts non-remission in major depression patients treated with citalopram in a 12-weeks follow up study. *J. Clin. Psychopharmacol.*, **23**, 563–7.

Arora, R. C. & Meltzer, H. Y. (1989). Serotonergic measures in the brains of suicide victims: 5-HT(2) binding sites in the frontal cortex of suicide victims and control subjects. *Am. J. Psychiatry*, **146**, 730–6.

Arranz, M. J., Collier, D., Sodhi, M. *et al.* (1995). Association between clozapine response and allelic variation in 5-HT2A receptor gene. *Lancet*, **346**, 281–2.

Arranz, M. J., Collier, D. A., Munro, J. *et al.* (1996). Analysis of a structural polymorphism in the 5-HT2A receptor and clinical response to clozapine. *Neurosci. Lett.* **217**, 177–8.

Arranz, M. J., Munro, J., Owen, M. J. *et al.* (1998). Evidence for association between polymorphisms in the promoter and coding regions of the 5-HT2A receptor gene and response to clozapine. *Mol. Psychiatry*, **3**, 61–6.

Basile, V. S., Ozdemir, V., Masellis, M. *et al.* (2000). A functional polymorphism of the cytochrome P450 1A2 (CYP1A2) gene: association with tardive dyskinesia in schizophrenia. *Mol. Psychiatry*, **5**, 410–17.

Basile, V. S., Masellis, M., Potkin, S. G. & Kennedy, J. L. (2002). Pharmacogenomics in schizophrenia: the quest for individualized therapy. *Hum. Mol. Genet.*, **11**, 2517–30.

Benjafield, A. V., Jeyasingam, C. L., Nyholt, D. R., Griffiths, L. R. & Morris, B. J. (1998). G protein beta3 subunit gene (GNB3) variant in causation of essential hypertension. *Hypertension*, **32**, 1094–7.

Bertilsson, L. (1995). Geographical/interracial differences in polymorphic drug oxidation: current state of knowledge of cytochrome P450 (CYP) 2D6 and 2C19. *Clin. Pharmacokinet.*, **29**, 192–209.

Bertilsson, L., Lou, Y. Q., Du, Y. L. *et al.* (1992). Pronounced differences between native Chinese and Swedish populations in the polymorphic hydroxylations of debrisoquin and S-mephenytoin. *Clin. Pharmacol. Ther.*, **51**, 338–97.

Bondy, B. & Zill, P. (2004). Pharmacogenetics and psychopharmacology. *Curr. Opin. Pharmacol.* **4**(1), 72–8.

Bondy, B., Baghai, T. C., Zill, P. *et al.* (2002). Combined action of the ACE D- and the G-protein beta3 T-allele in major depression: a possible link to cardiovascular disease? *Mol. Psychiatry*, **7**, 1120–6.

Bonisch, H. & Bruss, M. (1994). The noradrenaline transporter of the neuronal plasma membrane. *Ann. N.Y. Acad. Sci.*, **733**, 193–202.

Boularand, S., Darmon, M. C., Ganem, Y., Launay, J. M. & Mallet J. (1990). Complete coding sequence of human tryptophan hydroxylase. *Nucleic Acids Res.* **18**(14), 4257.

Burnet, P. W., Eastwood, S. L., Lacey, K. & Harrison, P. J. (1995). The distribution of 5-HT1A and 5-HT2A receptor mRNA in human brain. *Brain Res*, **675**, 157–68.

Chang, H. W., Yen, C. Y., Liu, S. Y., Singer, G. & Shih, I. E. M. (2002). Genotype analysis using human hair shaft. *Cancer Epidemiol. Biomarkers Prev.* **11**, 925–9.

Chen, K., Yang, W., Grimsby, J. & Shih, J. C. (1992). The human 5HT2A receptor is encoded by a multiple intron exon gene. *Brain Res. Mol. Brain Res.*, **14**, 20–6.

Choi, M. J., Kang, R. H., Ham, B. J., Jeong, H. Y. & Lee, M. S. (2005). Serotonin receptor 2A gene polymorphism (-1438A/G) and short-term treatment response to citalopram. *Neuropsychobiology*, **52**, 155–62.

Craddock, N. & Jones, I. (2001). Molecular genetics of bipolar disorder. *Br. J. Psychiatry Suppl.*, **41**, S128–S133.

Craig, S. P., Boularand, S., Darmon, M. C., Mallet, J. & Craig, I. W. (1991). Localization of human tryptophan hydroxylase (TPH) to chromosome 11p15.3-p14 by in situ hybridization. *Cytogenet. Cell Genet.*, **56**, 157–9.

Cusin, C., Serretti, A., Zanardi, R. *et al.* (2002). Influence of monoamine oxidase A and serotonin receptor 2A polymorphisms in SSRI antidepressant activity. *Int. J. Neuropsychopharmacol.*, **5**, 27–35.

Daniel, H. I. & Edeki, T. I. (1996). Genetic polymorphism of S-mephenytoin 4¢-hydroxylation *Psychopharmacol. Bull.*, **32**, 219–30.

DeBellis, M., Geracioti, T. & Altemus, M. (1993). Cerebrospinal fluid monoamine metabolites in fluoxetine treated patients with major depression and in healthy volunteers. *Biol. Psychiatry*, **33**, 636–41.

de Morais, S. M., Wilkinson, G. R., Blaisdell, J. *et al.* (1994). The major genetic defect responsible for the polymorphism of S-mephenytoin metabolism in humans. *J. Biol. Chem.*, **269**, 15419–22.

Del Zompo, M., Ardau, R., Palmas, M. A. *et al.* (1999). Lithium response: association study with two candidate genes. *Mol. Psychiatry*, **4**(1), S66–S67.

Dong, Y., Zhu, H., Sagnella, G. A. *et al.* (1999). Association between the C825T polymorphism of the G protein beta3- subunit gene and hypertension in blacks. *Hypertension*, **34**, 1193–6.

Durham, L. K., Webb, S. M., Milos, P. M., Clary, C. M. & Seymour, A. B. (2004). The serotonin transporter polymorphism, 5HTTLPR, is associated with a faster response time to sertraline in an elderly population with major depressive disorder. *Psychopharmacology*, **174**, 525–9.

Erdmann, J., Shimron-Abarbanell, D., Rietschel, M. *et al.* (1996). Systematic screening for mutations in the human serotonin-2A (5-HT$_{2A}$) receptor gene: identification of two naturally occurring receptor variants and association analysis in schizophrenia. *Hum. Genet.*, **97**, 614–19.

Ford, C. E., Skiba, N. P., Bae, H. *et al.* (1998). Molecular basis for interactions of G protein betagamma subunits with effectors. *Science*, **280**, 1271–4.

Glennon, R. A. & Dukat, M. (1995). Serotonin receptor subtypes. In F. E. Bloom and D. J. Kupfer, eds., *Psychopharmacology: The Fourth Generation of Progress*. New York, NY: Raven Press, pp. 1125–31.

Goldstein, J. A., Ishizaki, T., Chiba, K. *et al.* (1997). Frequencies of defective CYP2C19 alleles responsible for the mephenytoin poor metabolizer phenotype in various Oriental, Caucasian, Saudi Arabian and American black populations. *Pharmacogenetics*, **7**, 59–64.

Gonzalez, F. J. & Idle, J. R. (1994). Pharmacogenetic phenotyping and genotyping. Present status and future potential. *Clin. Pharmacokinet.*, **26**, 59–70.

Grof, P., Alda, M., Grof, E., Zvolsky, P. & Walsh, M. (1994). Lithium response and genetics of affective disorders. *J. Affect. Disord.*, **32**, 85–95.

Guttendorf, R. J. & Wedlund, P. J. (1992). Genetic aspects of drug disposition and therapeutics. *J. Clin. Pharmacology*, **32**, 107–17.

Ham, B. J., Lee, M. S., Lee, H. J. *et al.* (2005). No association between the tryptophan hydroxylase gene polymorphism and major depressive disorders and antidepressants response in a Korean population. *Psychiatr. Genet.*, **15**, 299–301.

Hamelin, B. A., Turgeon, J., Vallee, F. *et al.* (1996). The disposition of fluoxetine but not sertraline is altered in poor metabolizers of debrisoquin. *Clin. Pharmacol. Ther.*, **60**, 512–21.

Hamm, H. E. (1998). The many faces of G protein signaling. *J. Biol. Chem.*, **273**, 669–72.

Hegele, R. A., Anderson, C., Young, T. K. & Connelly, P. W. (1999). G-protein beta3 subunit gene splice variant and body fat distribution in Nunavut Inuit. *Genome Res.*, **9**, 972–7.

Heils, A., Teufel, A., Petri, S. *et al.* (1996). Allelic variation of human serotonin transporter gene expression. *J. Neurochem.*, **66**, 2621–4.

Hengstenberg, C., Schunkert, H., Mayer, B. *et al.* (2001). Association between a polymorphism in the G protein beta3 subunit gene (GNB3) with arterial hypertension but not with myocardial infarction. *Cardiovasc. Res.,* **49**: 820–7.

Hwu, H. G., Hong, C. W., Lee, Y. L. *et al.* (1998). Dopamine D4 receptor gene polymorphisms and neuroleptic response in schizophrenia. *Biol. Psychiatry*, **44**, 483–7.

Inaba, T., Nebert, D. W., Burchell, B. *et al.* (1995). Pharmacokinetics in clinical pharmacology and toxicology. *Cana. J. Physiol. Pharmacol.*, **73**, 331–8.

Johansson, I., Oscarson, M., Yue, Q. Y. *et al.* (1994). Genetic analysis of the Chinese cytochrome P-4502D locus: characterization of variant CYP2D6 gene present in subjects with diminished capacity for debrisoquine hydroxylation. *Mol. Pharmacol.* **46**, 452–9.

Joober, R., Benkelfat, C., Brisebois, K. *et al.* (1999). T102C polymorphism in the 5HT2A gene and schizophrenia: relation to phenotype and drug response variability. *J. Psych. Neurosci.*, **24**, 141–6.

Kaiser, R., Konneker, M., Henneken, M. *et al.* (2000). Dopamine D4 receptor 48-bp repeat polymorphism: no association with response to antipsychotic treatment, but association with catatonic schizophrenia. *Mol. Psychiatry*, **5**, 418–24.

Kalow, W. (1992). *Pharmacokinetics of Drug Metabolism.* New York, NY: Pergamon.

Kalow, W. & Bertilsson, L. (1994). Interethnic factors affecting drug response. *Adv. Drug Res.,* **25**, 1–53.

Kapitany, T., Meszaros, K., Lenzinger, E. *et al.* (1998). Genetic polymorphisms for drug metabolism (CYP2D6) and tardive dyskinesia in schizophr. *Schizophr. Res.*, **32**, 101–6.

Kim, C. H., Kim, H. S., Cubells, J. F., & Kim, K. S. (1999). A previously undescribed intron and extensive 5′upstream sequence, but not Phox2a-mediated transactivation, are necessary for high level cell type-specific expression of the human norepinephrine transporter gene. *J. Biol. Chem.,* **274**, 6507–18.

Kim, D. K., Lim, S. W., Lee, S. *et al.* (2000). Serotonin transporter gene polymorphism and antidepressants response. *Neuroreport*, **11**, 215–19.

Kohen, R., Metcalf, M. A., Khan, N. *et al.* (1996). Cloning, characterization and chromosomal localization of a human 5-HT6 serotonin receptor. *J. Neurochem.*, **66**, 47–56.

Kunugi, H., Kato, T., Fukuda, R. *et al.* (2002). Association study of C825T polymorphism of the G-protein beta3 subunit gene with schizophrenia and mood disorders. *J. Neural Transm.* **109**, 213–18.

Lake, C. R., Pickar, D., Ziegler, M. G. *et al.* (1982). High plasma norepinephrine levels in patients with major affective disorder. *Am. J. Psychiatry* **139**, 1315–18.

Lam, L. C. W., Garcia-Barcelo, M. M., Ungvari, G. S. *et al.* (2001). Cytochrome CYP2D6 genotyping and association with tardive dyskinesia in Chinese schizophrenic patients. *Pharmacopsychiatry*, **34**, 238–41.

Lane, H. Y., Chang, Y. C., Chiu, C. C. *et al.* (2002). Association of risperidone treatment response with a polymorphism in the 5-HT(2A) receptor gene. *Am. J. Psychiatry*, **159**, 1593–5.

Lee, H. J., Cha, J. H., Ham, B. J. *et al.* (2004). Association between a G-protein b3 subunit gene polymorphism and the symptomatology and treatment responses of major depressive disorders. *Pharmacogenomics J.* **4**, 29–33.

Lee, M. S., Lee, H. Y., Lee, H. J. & Ryu, S. H. (2004). Serotonin transporter promoter gene polymorphism and long-term outcome of antidepressants treatment. *Psychiatr. Genet.*, **14**, 111–15.

Lee, S. H., Lee, K. J., Lee, H. J. *et al.* (2005). Association between the 5-HT6 receptor C267T polymorphism and response to antidepressants treatment in major depressive disorder. *Psychiatry Clin. Neurosci.*, **59**, 140–5.

Lesch, K. P., Balling, U., Gross, J. *et al.* (1994). Organization of the human serotonin transporter gene. *J. Neural Transm. Gen. Sect.*, **95**, 157–62.

Lesch, K. P., Bengel, D., Heils, A. *et al.* (1996). Association of anxiety related traits with a polymorphism in the serotonin transporter gene regulatory region. *Science*, **274**, 1527–31.

Lin, C. H., Tsai, S. J., Yu, Y. W. *et al.* (1999). No evidence for association of serotonin-2A receptor variant (102T/C) with schizophrenia or clozapine response in a Chinese population. *Neuroreport* **10**, 57–60.

Lin, C. N., Tsai, S. J. & Hong, C. J. (2001a). Association analysis of a functional G protein beta3 subunit Gene polymorphism (C825T) in mood disorders. *Neuropsychobiology*, **44**, 118–21.

Lin, K. M. (2001b). Biological differences in depression and anxiety across races and ethnic groups, *J. Clin. Psychiatry*, **62** (13), 13–19.

Lin, K. M. & Cheung, F. (1999). Mental health issues for Asian Americans. *Psychiat. Serv.*, **50**, 774–80

Lin K. M. & Poland, R. E. (1995). Ethnicity, culture and psychopharmacology. In F. E. Bloom, & D. I. Kupfer, eds., *Psychopharmacology: The Fourth Generation of Progress.* New York, NY: Raven, pp.1907–17.

Lin, K. M., Poland, R. E. & Nakasaki, G. (eds.) (1993). *Psychopharmacology and Psychobiology of Ethnicity.* Washington, DC: American Psychiatric Press.

Lin, K. M., Poland, R. E., Wan, Y-J. Y., Smith, M. W. & Lesser, I. M. (1996). The evolving science of pharmacogenetics: clinical and ethnic perspectives. *Psychopharmacol. Bull.*, **32**, 205–17.

Lou, Y. C. (1990). Differences in drug metabolism polymorphism between Orientals and Caucasians. *Drug Metab. Rev.,* **22**, 451–75.

Maj, J., Bijak, M., Dziedzicka-Wasylewska, M. *et al.* (1996).  The effects of paroxetine given repeatedly on the 5-HT receptor subpopulations in the rat brain. *Psychopharmacology*, **127**, 73–82.

Malhotra, A., Goldman, D., Ozaki, N. *et al.* (1996a). Lack of association between polymorphisms in the 5-HT2A receptor gene and the antipsychotic response to clozapine. *Am. J. Psychiatry*, **153**, 1092–4.

Malhotra, A., Goldman, D., Ozaki, N. *et al.* (1996b). Clozapine response and the 5-HT2C Cys23Ser polymorphism. *Neuroreport*, **7**, 2100–2.

Malhotra, A. K., Goldman, D., Buchanan, R. W. *et al.* (1998). The dopamine D-3 receptor (DRD3) Ser-9Gly polymorphism and schizophrenia: a haplotype relative risk study and association with clozapine response. *Mol. Psychiatry*, **3**, 72–5.

Masellis, M., Basile, V. S., Ozdemir, V. *et al.* (2000). Pharmacogenetics of antipsychotic treatment: lessons learned from clozapine. *Biol. Psychiatry*, **47**, 252–66.

Masellis, M., Basile, V. S., Meltzer, H. Y. *et al.* (2001). Lack of association between the T–>C 267 serotonin 5-HT6 receptor gene (HTR6) polymorphism and prediction of response to clozapine in schizophrenia. *Schizophr. Res.*, **15**, 49–58.

Massana, J. (1998). Reboxetine versus fluoxetine: an overview of efficacy and tolerability. *J. Clin. Psychiatry*, **59**(14), 8–10.

Mendlewicz, J., Verbanck, P., Linkowski, P. & Wilmotte, J. (1978).  Lithium accumulation in erythrocytes of manic-depressive patients: an in vivo twin study. *Br. J. Psychiatry*, **133**, 436–44.

Meyer, J. H., Kapur, S., Eisfeld, B. & Brown, G. M. (2001). The effect of paroxetine on 5-HT(2A) receptors in depression: an [18F]setoperone PET imaging study. *Am. J. Psychiatry*, **158**, 78–86.

Meyer, U. A. (1994a). The molecular basis of genetic polymorphisms of drug metabolism. *J. Pharm. Pharmacol.*, **46**(1), 409–15.

Meyer, U. A. (1994b). Pharmacogenetics: the slow, therapid, and the ultrarapid. *Proc. Nat. Acad. Sci. USA*, **91**, 1983–4.

Meyer, U. A., Zanger, U. M., Grant, D. *et al.* (1990). Genetic polymorphisms of drug metabolism. *Adv. Drug Res.*, **19**, 197–241.

Minov, C., Baghai, T. C., Schule, C. *et al.* (2001).  Serotonin-2A-receptor and -transporter polymorphisms: lack of association in patients with major depression. *Neurosci. Lett.*, **303**, 119–22.

Monsma, F. J. Jr, Shen, Y., Ward, R. P., Hamblin, M. W. & Sibley, D. R. (1993).  Cloning and expression of a novel serotonin receptor with high affinity for tricyclic psychotropic drugs. *Mol. Pharmacol.*, **43**, 320–7.

Montgomery, S. A. (1994). Long-term treatment of depression. *Br. J. Psychiatry*, **26**(suppl), 31–6.

Murphy, G. M. Jr, Kremer, C., Rodrigues, H. E. & Schatzberg, A. F. (2003). Pharmacogenetics of antidepressant medication intolerance Am. J. Psychiatry*, **160**, 1830–5.

Nakamura, K., Goto, F., Ray, W. A. *et al.* (1985). Interethnic differences in genetic polymorphism of debrisoquine and mephenytoin hydroxylation between Japanese and Caucasian populations. *Clin. Pharmacol. Ther.*, **10**, 402–8.

Nielsen, D. A., Jenkins, G. L., Stefanisko, K. M., Jefferson, K. K. & Goldman, D. (1997). Sequence, splice site and population frequency distribution analyses of the polymorphic human tryptophan hydroxylase intron 7. *Brain Res. Mol. Brain Res.*, **45**, 145–8.

Nimgaonkar, V. L., Zhang, X. R., Brar, J. S. *et al.* (1996). 5-HT2 receptor gene locus: association with schizophrenia or treatment response not detected. *Psychiatr. Genet.*, **6**, 23–7.

Nöthen, M. M., Rietschel, M., Erd mann, J. *et al.* (1995). Genetic variation of the 5-HT2A receptor and response to clozapine. *Lancet*, **346**, 908–9.

Owens, M. J. (1997). Molecular and cellular mechanisms of antidepressants drugs. *Depress. Anxiety*, **4**, 153–9.

Phiel, C. J. & Klein, P. S. (2001). Molecular targets of lithium action. *Annu. Rev. Pharmacol. Toxicol.*, **41**, 789–813.

Pickar, D. & Rubinow, K. (2001) Pharmacogenomics of psychiatric disorders. *Trends Pharmacol. Sci.* **22**, 75–83.

Pollock, B. G., Ferrell, R. E., Mulsant, B. H. *et al.* (2000). Allelic variation in the serotonin transporter promoter affects onset of paroxetine treatment response in late-life depression. *Neuropsychopharmacol.*, **23**, 587–90.

Poolsup, N., Li Wan Po, A. & Knight, T. L. (2000). Pharmacogenetics and psychopharmacology. *J. Clin. Pharm. Ther.*, **25**, 197–200.

Porzgen, P., Bonisch, H. & Bruss, M. (1995). Molecular cloning and organization of the coding region of the human norepinephrine transporter gene. *Psychiatry*, **26**, 1279–83

Ramamoorthy, S., Bauman, A. L., Moore, K. R. *et al.* (1993). Antidepressants- and cocaine-sensitive human serotonin transporter: molecular cloning, expression, and chromosomal localization. *Proc. Natl. Acad. Sci. USA*, **90**, 2542–6.

Rao, P. A., Packer D., Gejman, P. V. *et al.* (1994). Allelic variation in the D4 dopamine receptor (DRD4) gene does not predict response to clozapine. *Arch. Gen. Psychiatry*, **51**, 912–17.

Rausch, J. L., Johnson, M. E., Fei, Y. J. *et al.* (2002). Initial conditions of serotonin transporter kinetics and genotype: influence on SSRI treatment trial outcome. *Biol. Psychiatry*, **51**, 723–32.

Reynolds, G. P., Zhang, Z. & Zhang, X. (2003). Polymorphism of the promoter region of the serotonin 5HT(2C) receptor gene and clozapine induced weight gain. *Am. J. Psychiatry*, **160**, 677–9.

Rietschel, M., Naber, D., Fimmers, R. *et al.* (1997). Efficacy and side effects of clozapine not associated with variation in the 5-HT2C receptor. *NeuroReport*, **8**, 1999–2003.

Roh, H. K., Dahl, M. L., Johansson, I. *et al.* (1996). Debrisoquine and S-mephenytoin hydroxylation phenotypes and genotypes in a Korean population. *Pharmacogenetics*, **6**, 441–7.

Rosskopf, D., Koch, K., Habich, C. *et al.* (2003). Interaction of Gbeta3s, a splice variant of the G-protein Gbeta3, with Ggamma- and Galpha-proteins. *Cell Signal*, **15**, 479–88.

Roth, B. L., Craigo, S. C., Choudhary, M. S. *et al.* (1994). Binding of typical and atypical antipsychotic agents to 5-hydroxytryptamine- 6 and 5-hydroxytryptamine-7 receptors. *J. Pharmacol. Exp. Ther.*, **268**, 1403–10.

Roy, A., Pickar, D., Dejong, J., Karoum, F. & Linnoila, M. (1998). Norepinephrine and its metabolites in cerebrospinal fluid, plasma and urine. Relationship to hypothalamic-pituitary-adrenal axis function in depression. *Arch. Gen. Psychiatry*, **45**, 849–57.

Sato, K., Yoshida, K., Takahashi, H. *et al.* (2002). Association between −1438G/A promoter polymorphism in the 5-HT(2A) receptor gene and fluvoxamine response in Japanese patients with major depressive disorder. *Neuropsychobiology*, **46**, 136–40.

Scates, A. C. & Doraiswamy, P. M. (2000). Reboxetine: a selective norepinephrine reuptake inhibitor for the treatment of depression. *Ann. Pharmacother.*, **34**, 1302–12.

Scharfetter, J., Chaudhry, H. R., Hornik, K. *et al.* (1999). Dopamine D3 receptor gene polymorphism and response to clozapine in schizophrenic Pakistani patients. *Eur. Neuropsychopharmacol.*, **10**, 17–20.

Seeman, P. & Vantol, H. H. M. (1994). Dopamine receptor pharmacology. *Trends Pharmacol. Sci.*, **15**, 264–70.

Serretti, A., Lilli, R., Lorenzi, C., Franchini, L. & Smeraldi, E. (1998). Dopamine receptor D3 gene and response to lithium prophylaxis in mood disorders. *Int. J. Neuropsychopharmacol.*, **1**, 125–9.

Serretti, A., Lilli, R., Lorenzi, C. *et al.* (1999). Dopamine receptor D2 and D4 genes, GABA(A) alpha- 1 subunit genes and response to lithium prophylaxis in mood disorders. *Psychiatry Res.*, **87**, 7–19.

Serretti, A., Lorenzi, C., Lilli, R. & Smeraldi, E. (2000). Serotonin receptor 2A, 2C, 1A genes and response to lithium prophylaxis in mood disorders. *J. Psychiatr. Res.*, **34**, 89–98.

Serretti, A., Zanardi, R., Cusin, C. *et al.* (2001a). Tryptophan hydroxylase gene associated with paroxetine antidepressants activity. *Eur. Neuropsychopharmacol.*, **11**, 375–80.

Serretti, A., Zanardi, R., Rossini, D. *et al.* (2001b). Influence of tryptophan hydroxylase and serotonin transporter genes on fluvoxamine antidepressants activity. *Mol. Psychiatry*, **6**, 586–92.

Serretti, A., Lorenzi, C., Cusin, C. *et al.* (2003). SSRIs antidepressants activity is influenced by Gbeta3 variants. *Eur. Neuropsychopharmacol.*, **13**, 117–22.

Serretti, A., Malitas, P. N., Mandelli, L. *et al.* (2004). Further evidence for a possible association between serotonin transporter gene and lithium prophylaxis in mood disorders. *Pharmacogenomics J.*, **4**(4), 267–73.

Shaikh, S., Collier, D. A., Sham, P. *et al.* (1995). Analysis of clozapine response and polymorphisms of the dopamine D4 receptor gene (DRD4) in schizophrenic patients. *Am. J. Med. Genet.*, **60**, 541–5.

Shaikh, S., Collier, D. A., Sham, P. C. *et al.* (1996). Allelic association between a Ser-9-Gly polymorphism in the dopamine D3 receptor gene and schizophrenia. *Hum. Genet.*, **97**, 714–19.

Shaldubina, A., Agam, G. & Belmaker, R. H. (2001). The mechanism of lithium action: state of the art, ten years later. *Prog. Neuropsychopharmacol. Biol. Psychiatry*, **25**, 855–66.

Siffert, W. (2003). G-protein beta3 subunit 825T allele and hypertension. *Curr. Hypertens. Rep.*, **5**, 47–53.

Siffert, W., Rosskopf, D., Siffert, G. *et al.* (1998). Association of a human G protein beta3 subunit variant with hypertension. *Nat. Genet.*, **18**, 45–8.

Siffert, W., Forster, P., Jockel, K. H. *et al.* (1999). Worldwide ethnic distribution of the G protein beta3 subunit 825T allele and its association with obesity in Caucasian, Chinese, and Black African individuals. *J. Am. Soc. Nephrol.*, **10**, 1921–30.

Skrebuhhova, T., Allikmets, L. & Matto, V. (1999). 5-HT2A receptors mediate the effects of antidepressants in the elevated plus-maze test but have a partial role in the forced swim test. *Med. Sci. Res.*, **27**, 277–80.

Sleight, A. J., Boess, F. G., Bos, M. & Bourson, A. (1998). The putative 5-ht6 receptor: localization and function. *Ann. N. Y. Acad. Sci.*, **861**, 91–6.

Smeraldi, E., Zanardi, R. & Benedetti, F. (1998). Polymorphism within the promoter of the serotonin transporter gene and antidepressants efficacy of fluvoxamine. *Mol. Psychiatry*, **3**, 508–11.

Smeraldi, E., Benedetti, F. & Zanardi, R. (2002). Serotonin transporter promoter genotype and illness recurrence in mood disorders. *Eur. Neuropsychopharmacol.* **12**, 73–5.

Smith, M. W. & Mendoza, R. P. (1996). Ethnicity and pharmacogenetics. *Mt. Sinai. J. Med.*, **63**, 285–90.

Sodhi, M. S., Arranz, M. J., Curtis, D. *et al.* (1995). Association between clozapine response and allelic variation in the 5-HT2C receptor gene. *Neuroreport*, **7**, 169–72.

Spurlock, G., Helis, A., Holmas, P. *et al.* (1998). A family based association study of T 102C polymorphism in 5HT2A and schizophrenia plus identification of new polymorphisms in the promoter. *Mol. Psychiatry*, **3**, 42–9.

Szot, P., Ashliegh, E. A., Kohen, R. *et al.* (1993). Norepinephrine transporter mRNA is elevated in the locus coeruleus following short- and long-term desipramine treatment. *Brain Res.*, **618**, 308–12.

Turecki, G., Grof, P., Grof, E. *et al.* (2001). Mapping susceptibility genes for bipolar disorder: a pharmacogenetic approach based on excellent response to lithium. *Mol. Psychiatry*, **6**, 570–8.

Veith, R. C., Lewis, N., Linares, O. A. *et al.* (1994). Sympathetic nervous system activity in major depression. *Arch. Gen. Psychiatry*, **51**, 411–22.

Virchow, S., Ansorge, N., Rosskopf, D., Rubben, H. & Siffert, W. (1999). The G protein beta3 subunit splice variant Gbeta3-s causes enhanced chemotaxis of human neutrophils in response to interleukin-8. *Naunyn- Schmiedeberg's Arch. Pharmacol.*, **360**, 27–32.

Vogt, I. R., Shimron-Abarbanell, D., Neidt, H. *et al.* (2000). Investigation of the human serotonin 6 [5HT6] receptor gene in bipolar affective disorder and schizophrenia. *Am. J. Med. Genet.*, **96**, 217–21.

Wang, J. H., Liu, Z. Q., Wang, W. *et al.* (2001). Pharmacokinetics of sertraline in relation to genetic polymorphism of CYP2C19. *Clin. Pharmacol. Ther.*, **70**, 42–7.

Ward, R. P., Hamblin, M. W., Lachowicz, J. E. *et al.* (1995). Localization of serotonin subtype 6 receptor messenger RNA in the rat brain by in situ hybridization histochemistry. *Neuroscience*, **64**, 1105–11.

Weinshilboum, R. (2003). Inheritance and drug response. *N. Engl. J. Med.*, **384**, 529–37.

Wu, W. H., Huo, S. J., Cheng, C. Y., Hong, C. J. & Tsai, S. J. (2001). Association study of the 5-HT (6) receptor polymorphism (C267T) and symptomatology and antidepressant response in major depressive disorders. *Neuropsychobiology*, **44**, 172–5.

Yates, M., Leake, A., Candy, J. M. *et al.* (1990). 5HT2 receptor changes in major depression. *Biol. Psychiatry*, **27**, 489–96.

Yatham, L. N., Liddle, P. F. & Dennie, J. (1999). Decrease in brain serotonin 2 receptor binding in patients with major depression following desipramine treatment: a positron emission tomography study with fluorine-18-labeled setoperone. *Arch. Gen. Psychiatry*, **56**, 705–11.

Yoshida, K., Ito, K., Sato, K. *et al.* (2002a). Influence of the serotonin transporter gene-linked polymorphic region on the antidepressants response to fluvoxamine in Japanese depressed patients. *Prog. Neuropsychopharmacol. Biol. Psychiatry*, **26**, 383–6.

Yoshida, K., Naito, S., Takahashi, H. *et al.* (2002b). Monoamine oxidase: a gene polymorphism, tryptophan hydroxylase gene polymorphism and antidepressants response to fluvoxamine in Japanese patients with major depressive disorder. *Prog. Neuropsychopharmacol. Biol. Psychiatry*, **26**, 1279–83.

Yoshida, K., Takahashi, H., Higuchi, H. *et al.* (2004). Prediction of antidepressants response to milnacipran by norepinephrine transporter gene polymorphisms. *Am. J. Psychiatry*, **161**(9), 1575–80.

Yoshioka, M., Matsumoto, M., Togashi, H. & Mori, K. (1998). Central distribution and function of 5-HT6 receptor subtype in the rat brain. *Ann. N.Y. Acad. Sci.*, **861**, 244.

Yu, Y. W., Tsai, S. J., Lin, C. H. *et al.* (1999). Serotonin-6 receptor variant (C267T) and clinical response to clozapine. *Neuroreport*, **10**, 1231–3.

Yu, Y. W., Tsai, S. J., Chen, T. J., Lin, C. H. & Hong, C. J. (2002). Association study of the serotonin transporter promoter polymorphism and symptomatology and antidepressants response in major depressive disorders. *Mol. Psychiatry*, **7**, 1115–19.

Zanardi, R., Benedetti, F., Di Bella, D., Catalano, M. & Smeraldi, E. (2000). Efficacy of paroxetine in depression is influenced by a functional polymorphism within the promoter of the serotonin transporter gene. *J. Clin. Psychopharmacol.*, **20**, 105–7.

Zill, P., Baghai, T. C., Zwanzger, P. *et al.* (2000). Evidence for an association between a G-protein beta3-gene variant with depression and response to antidepressants treatment. *Neuroreport*, **11**, 1893–7.

Zill, P., Engel, R., Baghai, T. C. *et al.* (2002). Identification of a naturally occurring polymorphism in the promoter region of the norepinephrine transporter and analysis in major depression. *Neuropsychopharmacol.*, **26**, 489–93.

# 6

# Variation in psychotropic responses in the Chinese population

Tian-Mei Si

## Psychopharmacotherapy in the Chinese population

Traditional medicine, especially herbal medicine and acupuncture, has a long history in China. Included in the voluminous classic literature of traditional Chinese medicine are specific acupuncture procedures and a large number of herbal formulas that have been regarded as useful for the treatment of mental disorders. Although most of these methods have not yet been examined with rigorous clinical trials, it does appear that, in general, they are likely to be effective in the treatment of mood disorders, but not psychotic disorders. Systematic settings to provide care for the severely mentally ill started in late nineteenth century. The first European styled mental hospital was established in Guangzhou, China, in 1898. Gradually more mental hospitals were established in other large cities in China. However, until the introduction of chlorpromazine in the 1950s, therapeutic options were extremely limited, and traditional Chinese medicine therapy, insulin coma, and electro-convulsive therapy (ECT) were commonly used for the treatment of severely disturbed patients.

As is true worldwide, the arrival of the phenothiazines in the 1950s heralded a new era for the treatment of psychotic disorders in China. The earliest antipsychotic medications used included rauwolfiae, reserpine, promazine, and acetylpromazine. In 1956, domestic chlorpromazine was produced in Shanghai. Based on open clinical trials and descriptive clinical case observations, the clinical profiles of these potent agents, including their efficacy and tolerability, were established in the Chinese populations. In the subsequent two decades, however, they were gradually replaced in clinical practice by other newer domestic psychotropics considered to belong to the same class of neuroleptics with similar psychopharmacologic characteristics, and chemical structures. These were later called the

*Ethno-psychopharmacology: Advances in Current Practice*, eds. C. H. Ng, K.-M. Lin, B. S. Singh and E. Y. K. Chiu. Published by Cambridge University Press. © C. H. Ng, K.-M. Lin, B. S. Singh and E. Y. K. Chiu 2008.

typical antipsychotics, and included chlorpromazine, perphenazine, trifluoper-azine, fluphenazine, pipothiazine, chlorprothixene, haloperidol, penfluridol, sul-pride, and thioridazine. At the time, an implicit belief was that the therapeutic antipsychotic properties and adverse motor effects of these drugs were inextricably linked. Side effects such as the acute extrapyramidal symptoms (EPS), includ-ing Parkinsonism, dystonia, and akathisia, often are persistent and troublesome. Tardive dyskinesia (TD) is even worse, and the symptoms often are irreversible. Extrapyramidal symptoms and a host of other side effects contribute to the prob-lems of stigmata already plaguing schizophrenic patients, and to breakdowns in doctor–patient relationships, as well as treatment non-adherence, which in turn increases the risk of relapse and rehospitalization.

Clozapine treatment represented a miracle in the psychiatric care in China. Begin-ning in the 1970s, domestic clozapine was developed in China. Since then, it has been widely used throughout the country because of its proven superior effects on both the positive and negative symptoms, and also because of its low risks for EPS. As shown in a pharmaco-epidemiological investigation in 2002, clozapine was the first medication used by most psychiatrists to treat schizophrenia in both outpa-tient and inpatient settings in China. Even as the prototype atypical antipsychotic, clozapine is, however, not expensive in China. This consideration, combined with its excellent and broad-spectrum efficacy as well as a low risk for EPS, contributed towards clozapine's continuing popularity as a first-line antipsychotic in China.

Risperidone was launched in China in 1997. Following that, other atypical medi-cation including olanzapine and quetiapine were introduced in the market in 1999 and 2000, respectively. These were followed by the development of generic arip-iprazole and ziprasadone in 2005 and 2006, respectively. Brand-name aripiprazole and ziprasadone will also be launched in 2007 in China.

Iproniazid and pheniprazine were two of the earliest antidepressants to become available in China. In the 1960s, tricyclic antidepressants (TCAs) including doxe-pine, amitriptyline, and imipramine were introduced in clinical practice. Their indications included depression and anxiety from the beginning. This, however, led to the fading out of monoamine oxidase inhibitors (MAOIs) (iproniazid and pheniprazine) from clinical practice, because of their perceived high risks in induc-ing serotonin syndrome, as well as dietary restrictions. Since the 1990s, many novel antidepressants, including selective serotonin re-uptake inhibitors (SSRIs), sero-tonin and noradrenaline re-uptake inhibitors (SNRIs), and noradrenergic and spe-cific serotonergic antidepressants (NaSSAs), have been launched in China, with escitalopram as the most recent to be marketed in China, which was launched in 2007. The pharmaco-epidemiological study conducted in 2002 showed that SSRIs had already become the first-line medication to treat the depression and anxiety spectrum disorders, accounting for 42% of all antidepressant treatments.

**Table 6.1** The chronology of the development of psychotropics in China

| Time | Drugs | Indications |
|------|-------|-------------|
| 1956 | Chlorpromazine, Reserpine, Promazine, Acetylpromazine Perphenazine, Trifluoperazine, Fluphenazine | Psychosis |
| 1960–1979 | Pipothiazine, Chlorprothixene, Haloperidol, Penfluridol, Clozapine, Sulpride, Thioridazine | |
| | Doxepine, Amitriptyline, Imipramine, Iproniazid, Pheniprazine | Depression and anxiety |
| | Lithium | Mania |
| 1980–1990 | Fluphenazine decanoate, Pipothiazine palmitate, Haloperidol decanoate, Flupenthixol decanoate, Clopenthixol decanoate | Psychosis |
| | Clormipramine | Depression, anxiety, OCD |
| | Carbamazepine, Sodium valproate | Mania |
| 1991–2000 | Risperidone, Olanzapine, Quetiapine (Seroquel) | Psychosis |
| | Maprotiline, Moclobemide, Mianserin, Fluoxetine (Prozac), Paroxetine, Sertraline, Fluvoxamine, Citalopram, Venlafaxin (generic IR formulation and the brand Venlafaxine XR), Mirtazapine, Flupentixol-melitracen (Deanxit), Tianeptine, Extract of St. John's Wort, Buspirone | Depression and anxiety |
| 2001–present | Generic aripiprazole, ziprasadone and bupropion | Psychosis |
| | Escitalopram (lexpro), Tandospirone | Depression and anxiety |
| | Atypical antipsychotics (Risperidone) | Mania |

Introduced in clinical practice in the 1960s, lithium was the first mood stabilizer to be used in China. This was followed by carbamazepine and sodium valproate. For many years, these were the only treatment options available as mood stabilizers. Although lamotrigine was approved for maintenance treatment of bipolar I disorder in 2003 by FDA (Food and Drug Administration) in the USA, this indication has not yet been approved by the Chinese authorities. At present, only one atypical antipsychotic drug, risperidone, has been approved for treating acute mania (February 2005 by SFDA [State Food and Drug Administration]) in China (see Table 6.1).

The past two decades also have witnessed a steady progress towards an increasing level of sophistication in the study designs of clinical studies in China, ranging from case observations to multicenter comparison studies. The first double-blind comparison study in the field of psychiatry was conducted in China in 1984, for the comparison of the efficacy and safety of penfluridol and fluphenazine decanoate in treating patients with schizophrenia. During the past 20 years, clinical trials and other clinical studies have become increasingly more standardized and scientifically rigorous, and many of the studies have been sponsored by the SFDA or have been part of international collaborative efforts.

## Variations in the pharmacokinetics and pharmacodynamics of psychotropics in the Chinese population

Ethic variations in medication responses include differences in therapeutic responses and susceptibility to adverse effects. Such differences are attributable mostly to two aspects, the variation of enzyme activities for the metabolism of medications, and variations of the drugs' interactions with target binding sites.

Five cytochrome P450 enzymes are responsible for most of the metabolism of the majority of psychotropic drugs in use. These are: CYP1A2, CYP3A4, CYP2C9, CYP2C19, and CYP2D6. Ethnic variations in the activities of these enzymes, either due to genetic or non-genetic reasons, are often prominent. In the following, some of the most important findings relevant to the Chinese population will be briefly summarized.

CYP2D6 is one of the most important drug-metabolizing enzymes responsible for the metabolism of many of the commonly used antidepressants and neuroleptics. The CYP2D6 gene is highly polymorphic with more than 70 allelic variants, of which *CYP2D6*10* is particularly important for the Orientals because it is highly prevalent (allele frequency around 70%) and is by and large population specific. *CYP2D6*10* encodes the CYP2D6 enzyme with lower activities, leading to slower clearance of drugs dependent on this enzyme for metabolism. At the same time, with a much lower rate of allele frequency for *CYP2D6*4* encoding dysfunctional enzymes, Orientals were much less likely to be poor metabolizers (PMs). In contrast to the PM rate of 5–9% in Caucasians, approximately only 1% of the Chinese are PMs. However, China is a big country with populations belonging to diverse nationalities and ancestral backgrounds. This is reflected in the prevalence of the rate of PM of CYP2D6, ranging from 0%–1% for the Hans, 1.52% for the Zangs, 0.63% for the Urghurs, 0.81% for Mongolians, 0.8% for the Tongs, and 0% for the Miaos (Shu, Y. *et al.*, 2001; Li, G. C., *et al.*, 2005). CYP2D6 with identical pharmacological and molecular properties was also identified in the brain, and is functionally associated with the dopamine transporter and shares similarities in substrates and inhibitors, suggesting a role in dopaminergic neurotransmission. A study conducted in China (Fu, Y. *et al.*, 2006a; Huang, Y. *et al.*, 2002b) found that the polymorphism of C/T188 in CYP2D6 exon 1( *10) was associated with the clinical efficacy of risperidone in treating the schizophrenia. However, no such association was found in other studies also conducted in Chinese patients (Wang, B. *et al.*, 2004). In addition, several studies also examined the polymorphism of CYP2D6 and the therapeutic effects of antidepressants in Chinese populations (Liu, S. Q. *et al.*, 2000; Lin, J. R. *et al.*, 2002a, 2002b). The results did not show the association between the polymorphism of CYP2D6 and the efficacy of fluoxetine and paroxetine in treating patients with depression. Other studies found the *CYP2D6\*10* and the C163A polymorphism of the CYP1A2 gene may be associated with neuroleptic drug-induced TD in Chinese patients with schizophrenia (Fu, Y. *et al.*, 2006a; Fu, Y. *et al.*, 2006b).

CYP2C19 is also responsible for the metabolism of many psychotropic drugs. There are marked inter-racial differences in the frequency of the PM phenotype, ranging from 2–5% in Caucasians to 18–23% in the Asian populations. A number of studies have focused on the *CYP2C19* polymorphisms in various Chinese populations (Wu, M. L. *et al.*, 2005; Zhang, S. *et al.*, 2002; Huang, Y. *et al.*, 2002a). They revealed that two defective alleles, designated as *CYP2C19\*2(m1)* and *CYP2C19\*3(m2)*, are responsible for the genetic defects responsible for the PMs in China. Diazepam, sodium valproate, amitriptyline and citalopram are mainly metabolized by CYP2C19 (Liu, Z. Q. *et al.*, 2001; Chen, L. X. *et al.*, 2005; Fu, Q. L. *et al.*, 2005; Qi, X. I. *et al.*, 2004; Si, T. M. *et al.*, 2006). Some studies have shown that PMs of *CYP2C19* experienced slower metabolism of these drugs in Chinese patients with depression and seizure disorders (Qi, X. I. *et al.*, 2004; Chen, J. *et al.*, 2005). The *CYP2C19* also shows the gene dose effect on drug metabolism (Si, T. M. *et al.*, 2006). The $AUC_{0-t}$, $AUC_{0-\infty}$ of citalopram or escitalopram in subjects with heterozygote of PM (wt/m1 or wt/m2) are lower than the subjects of PMs, but higher than that of Ems (Si, T. M. *et al.*, 2006].

CYP1A2 is affected by environmental factors more than by heredity (Tantcheva-Poor *et al.*, 1999). The frequencies of different alleles appear to be similar between Caucasians and Oriental populations. The activity of CYP1A2 is different between the different regions of China (Shu, Y. *et al.*, 2001; Han, X. M. *et al.*, 2000). Fluvoxamine is a potent inhibitor of CYP1A2. Fluvoxamine can inhibit the N-demethylate metabolism of imipramine, clozapine, and clomipramine in Chinese populations (Li, F. *et al.*, 2004; Wang, C. Y. *et al.*, 2003; Yang, C. *et al.*, 2002; Wang, C. Y. *et al.*, 2000; Zhu, B. *et al.*, 1999; Wu, Z. L. *et al.*, 1998; Xu, Z. H. *et al.*, 1996). Similarly, CYP3A4 and CYP2C9 also play significant roles in the metabolism of many psychotropic drugs (e.g., olanzapine, clozapine, and quetiapine). When these medications are combined with inducers or inhibitors of CYP3A4, such as carbamazepine, a CYP3A4 enzyme inducer, the dose of these drugs needs to be adjusted. Since many of these enzyme inducers and inhibitors are natural substances that may differentially affect different populations.

Psychotropic drugs, including antidepressants, anti-anxiety agents, antipsychotic agents, mood stabilizers, and other agents act on the central nervous system. Variations in the genes encoding putative therapeutic targets of these medications likely influence their pharmacodynamic responses. Many such studies have focused on the susceptibility genes for schizophrenia, depression and related mood disorders, anxiety disorders including obsessive compulsive disorder (OCD), and panic disorders. Different approaches have been utilized for such studies, including genomic scanning or some target neurotransmitter systems, including $D_{1-5}$, $5\text{-}HT_{1A}$, transporters, and monoamine oxidax (MAO). DRD4 gene polymorphism (48bp VNTR) may be associated with quantitative characteristics of schizophrenia in Chinese, especially thought disturbance and conceptual derangement, patients with genotype of long variant may develop more severe symptoms (Zhao, A. L. et al., 2005). S/S genotype of 5-HTTLPR might be the susceptible gene (Wang, X. X. et al., 2004). Some of such studies also evaluated these susceptibility genes for the prediction of the efficacy or adverse effects of psychotropic drugs. Serotonin 2A receptor gene polymorphism (T102C$\propto$A-1438G) might be associated with TD in Chinese chronic male schizophrenia (Zhang, X. B. et al., 2005) and the effects of risperidone in treatment schizophrenia (Wang, Y. H. et al., 2006). Depressive patients with L/L genotype of 5-HTTLPR might be more responsive to the treatment of SSRIs (Wang, X. X. et al., 2004).

## The clinical responses of psychotropic drugs in Chinese populations

Data from randomized, controlled multicenter trials in native Chinese populations showed that the response rates (defined as reduction of PANSS scores of more than 50% from baseline) for atypical antipsychotic drugs, including olanzapine, clozapine, risperidone and quetiapine, were 64.0–73.3% after short-term treatment (6 weeks), as compared to rates ranging from 42.9% to 60% with haloperidol treatment) (An, B. F. et al., 2006; Li, C. et al., 2005; Liu, W. B. et al., 2004; Kong, Q. M. et al., 2003; Wang, G. et al., 2004; Zhou, M. et al., 2002; Hou, Y. Z. et al., 2001). Response rates (defined as HAM-D score reduction of more than 50% from the baseline) for the SSRIs, SNRIs, or NaSSA were 78–91%, and the remission (defined as HAMD $\leq$7) rate was 55–69% (Jiang, R. H. et al., 2006; Chen, J. D. et al., 2006; Shen, Y. F. et al., 2005; Yao, G. Z. et al., 1997; Si, T. M. et al., 2005a; Si, T. M. & Shu, L. 2006). Clinical trials also showed a response rate of 79% after four weeks of risperidone treatment (mean dosage 4.6 mg/day) for bipolar I disorder, as compared to 76% with haloperidol (8.0 mg/day) (Zang, S. et al., 2006).

Psychopharmaco-epidemiology investigation in China in 2002 showed that the first six antipsychotic drugs used for schizophrenia were clozapine, risperidone, sulpride, chlorpromazine, perphenazine, and haloperidol. The mean chlorpromazine equivalent dosage was 300 ± 201 mg/day for the outpatients and 409 ± 274 mg/day for the inpatients. 6.5% of the patients were treated with depot antipsychotic. More than two thirds of the patients were treated with monopharmacy. Among these patients with monopharmacy, 43.0% of them were treated with typical neuroleptics and 31.6% were treated with clozapine. These patients were more likely to be older, with a chronic course of illness, and experiencing disorganized speech and behaviors. In contrast, patients treated with atypical antipsychotics were more likely to be younger, with a shorter course of illness, and experiencing more delusions or hallucinations that could be either mood congruent or incongruent (Si, T. M. *et al.*, 2003; Si, T. M. *et al.*, 2004a). In terms of antidepressants, 44.5% of the patients with depression were treated with SSRIs. Patients with prominent symptoms of excitement or agitation were typically treated concomitantly with benzodiazepines. The most common adverse effects induced by antidepressants were vegetative nervous system symptoms including dry mouth and constipation; these were followed by nervous system symptoms including sedation, akathisia, and tremor. Patients treated with TCAs often experienced constipation, dry mouth, postural hypotension, tremor, salivation, and weight gain. Most patients treated with novel antidepressants developed sexual dysfunction, insomnia, or agitation (Si, T. M. *et al.*, 2004b). The treatment of bipolar disorder was different. Polypharmacy was very common (more than 80%), most often with mood stabilizers and atypical antipsychotic agents. 80.2% of patients with bipolar depression were treated with antidepressants alone, or in combination with mood stabilizers (Si, T. M. *et al.*, 2005b).

## Concluding remarks

In summary, modern psychopharmacotherapy in China has a history of nearly 50 years. The available data showed that although in many ways the progress of the field in China paralleled the worldwide trend, there were also unique patterns and approaches that have emerged from the Chinese experiences. Such differences in psychotropic responses are partially determined by ethic variations in the activities of the drug-metabolizing enzymes as well as variations in these drugs' target binding sites. Further elucidation of such influences is crucial for the rational use of these powerful and valuable therapeutic armamentaria in an increasingly evidence-based and individually tailored manner, taking into consideration each patient's socio-cultural and ethnic background. With its large and diverse populations, China has and will continue to play an important role in contributing significantly towards such goals.

## REFERENCES

An, B. F., Zhang, M. L. & Qi, S. G. (2006). Comparative study between the effect of olanzapine and quetiapine in first-episode schizophrenia. *Chinese Journal of Clinical Psychiatry*, **16**(2), 84–5.

Chen, J., Lu, Z., Jiang, S. D. *et al.* (2005). Association between polymorphism in the cytochrome P450 enzymes 1A2 2C19 gene and treatment-resistant depression. *Shanghai Archive of Psychiatry*, **17**(2), 95–8.

Chen, J. D., Guo, X. F., Xue, Z. M. *et al.* (2006). A randomized and double blind positive control clinical trial of bupropion SR for the treatment of depression. *Chinese Journal of New Drugs*, **15**(5), 379–82.

Chen, L. X., Wang, Z. G., Ai, M. *et al.* (2005). Effect of CYP2C19 genotypes on demethylation of amitriptyline in Chinese patients with depression. *Chinese Journal of Nervous and Mental Diseases*, **31**(1), 33–6.

Fu, Q. L., Huang, F., Wu, D. Z. *et al.* (2005). Analyses of the phenotype polymorphism of cytochrome CYP2C19 in Chinese Han. *Chinese Journal of New Drugs*, **14**(4), 461–4.

Fu, Y., Fan, C. H., Zhao, Z. H. *et al.* (2006a). Association of CYP2D6 gene C188T polymorphism with tardive dyskinesia (TD) in Chinese patients with schizophrenia. *Chinese Journal of Behavioral Medicine*, **15**(1), 36–7.

Fu, Y., Fan, C. H., Deng, H. H. *et al.* (2006b). Association of CYP2D6 and CYP1A2 gene polymorphism with tardive dyskinesia in Chinese schizophrenic patients. *Acta Pharmacol Sin*, **27**(3), 328–32.

Han, X. M., Chen, X. P., Wu, Q. N. *et al.* (2000). G-2964A and C734A genetic polymorphisms of CYP1A2 in Chinese population. *Acta Pharmacologica Sinica*, **21**, 1031–4.

Hou, Y. Z., Guo, J. H., Zhou, F. *et al.* (2001). The double-blind study of risperidone and haloperidal in the treatment of schizophrenia. *Shanghai Archive of Psychiatry*, **13**(3), 149–51.

Huang, Y., Ding, H., Wang, W. Z. *et al.* (2002a). The genetic polymorphisms of CYP2C19 and CYP2C9 in Chinese patients with epilepsy. *Journal of Chinese Clinical Medicine*, **3**(20), 4–6.

Huang, Y., Liu, X. H., Xu, K. *et al.* (2002b). Association study of cytochrome P450 2D6 gene polymorphism and therapeutic response to risperidone in Chinese subjects with schizophrenia. *Journal of Chinese Psychiatry*, **35**(2), 103–6.

Jiang, R. H., Shu, L., Zhang, H. Y. *et al.* (2006). A phase II randomized double blind multi-centers and parallel control clinical trial for bupropion SR in the treatment of depressive disorders. *Chinese Journal of New Drugs*, **15**(2), 128–31.

Kong, Q. M., Si, T. M. & Shu, L. (2003). The effects of olanzapine on body weight liver functions blood sugar and cholesterol level. *Chinese Journal of New Drugs*, **12**(10), 847–9.

Li, C., Chu, S. Y., Lin, Z. *et al.* (2005). A controlled study of olanzapine and haloperidol in the treatment of the acute phrase of schizophrenia. *Shanghai Archive of Psychiatry*, **17**(5), 275–7.

Li, F., Jiang, K. D., Jiang, S. D. *et al.* (2004). Novel mutation of the cytochrome P450 1A2 gene associated with the clinical response to clozapine in Chinese schizophrenic patients. *Shanghai Archive of Psychiatry*, **16**(3), 136–40.

Li, G. C., Yang, J., Chen, Z. G. *et al.* (2005). Expression of cytokine and gene polymorphism of CYP2D6 in Han Urghur and Hasake nationality in China. *Chinese Journal of Pharmaceuticals*, **40**(17), 1330–2.

Lin, J. R., Hou, J., Lu, X. Q. *et al.* (2002a). The relationship between the polymorphism of cytochrome P4502D6 and clinical response of paroxetine in Chinese. *The Chinese Journal of Clinical Pharmacology*, **18**(1), 22–5.

Lin, J. R., Zhen, D. *et al.* (2002b). Correlation between polymorphism of cytochrome P450 2D6 gene and clinical response to fluoxetine. *Journal of Chinese Psychiatry*, **35**(1), 18–21.

Liu, S. Q., Wang, J. H. & Zhou, H. H. (2000). Pharmacokinetics of fluoxetine and its effects on cytochrome P450 isoenzymes. *Acta Pharmacologica Sinica*, **16**(6), 618–20.

Liu, W. B., Li, H. C., Zhen, L. L. *et al.* (2004). A controlled study on olanzapine and clozapine in the treatment of the acute phase of schizophrenia. *Shanghai Archive of Psychiatry*, **16**(5), 282–4.

Liu, Z. Q., Shu, Y., Huang, S. L. *et al.* (2001). Effects of CYP2C19 genotype and CYP2C9 on fluoxetine N-demethylation in human liver microsomes. *Acta Pharmacologica Sinica*, **22**: 85–90.

Qi, X. l., Huang, Y., Wang, Y. Q. *et al.* (2004). Association of plasma sodium phenytoin concentration with CYP2C19 gene polymorphism. *Chinese Journal of New Drugs*, **13**(10), 922–5.

Shen, Y. F., Li, H. F., Ma, C. *et al.* (2005). Comparison of reboxetine with fluoxetine in treatment of depression:a randomized double-blind multicenter study. *Chinese Journal of New Drugs and Clinical Remedies*, **24**(8), 619–23.

Shu, Y., Cheng, Z. N., Liu, Z. Q. *et al.* (2001). Interindividual variations in levels and activities of cytochrome P-450 in liver microsomes of Chinese subjects. *Acta Pharmacologica Sinica*, **22**(3), 283–8.

Si, T. M. & Shu, L. (2006). Open-label study the effects of venlafaxine-XR in the treatment of depression. *Chinese Journal of Nervous and Mental Diseases*, **32**(1), 69–71.

Si, T. M., He, Y. L., Zhou, R. Y. *et al.* (2003). Psychotropics prescription pattern for the inpatients with schizophrenia. *Journal of Chinese Mental Health*, **17**(10), 705–7.

Si, T. M., Shu, L., Yu, X. *et al.* (2004a). Antipsychotic drug patterns of schizophrenia in China: a cross sectional study. *Chinese Journal of Psychiatry*, **37**(3), 152–5.

Si, T. M., Shu, L., Yu, X. *et al.* (2004b). Pharmacoepidemiological investigation on patients with depression in China. *Chinese Journal of Nervous and Mental Diseases*, **30**(2), 81–4.

Si, T. M., Shu, L., Yu, X. *et al.* (2005a). The efficacy and safety of citalopram in treatment of depression: a multi-center open-label study. *Chinese Journal of Psychiatry*, **38**(4), 222–6.

Si, T. M., Shu, L., Yu, X. *et al.* (2005b). A cross-sectional study on medication treatment patterns of bipolar disorder in China. *Chinese Journal of Psychiatry*, **38**(3), 165–9.

Si, T. M., Yang, Q., Liu, Y. *et al.* (2006). The relationship between the genetic polymorphism of CYP P450 2C19 and the pharmacokinetics of escitalopram in Chinese volunteers. *Chinese Journal of New Drugs*, **15**(15), 1296–9.

Tantcheva-Poor, I., Zaigler, M., Rietbrock, S. *et al.* (1999). Estimation of cytochrome P450 CYP1A2 activity in 863 healthy Caucasians using a saliva-based caffeine test. *Pharmacogenetics*, **9**, 131–44.

Wang, B., Yang, X. M., Jiang, S. D. *et al.* (2004). Genetic analysis of the cytochrome P450–2D6(CYP2D6) locus: screening influence of risperidone on clinical outcomes in schizophrenia. *Shanghai Archive of Psychiatry*, **16**(4), 199–202.

Wang, C. Y., Zhao, J. P., Chen, Y. G. *et al.* (2000). The pharmacokinetics of clozapine correlated with a caffeine test. *Journal of Chinese Psychiatry*, **33**(1), 16–18.

Wang, C. Y., Li, W. B., Zhai, Y. M. *et al.* (2003). Inhibition of olanzapine metabolism in vivo by fluvoxamine: a pharmacokinetic study in man. *Journal of Chinese Psychiatry*, **36**(1), 3–6.

Wang, G., Cai, Z. J., Wang, L. F. *et al.* (2004). A multicenter study of risperidone treatment for acute agitation in patients with schizophrenia. *Journal of Chinese Psychiatry*, **37**(2), 88–91.

Wang, X. X., Mu, J. S. & Wang, S. H. (2004). Association study of serotonin transporter gene polymorphism and depression. *Chinese Journal of Clinical Psychiatry*, **14**(4), 195–7.

Wang, Y. H., Shi, Z. Y., Zhao, G. Q. *et al.* (2006). Association between 5-HT2A receptor gene polymorphism and risperidone treatment response in the first episode (drug-naive) Chinese patients with schizophrenia. *Chinese Journal of Nervous and Mental Diseases*, **32**(4), 294–9.

Wu, M. L., Wu, X. H. & Chen, S. C. (2005). Study on tissue distribution difference of cytochrome P450 2C19 in Chinese population Han. *Journal of Chinese Pharmaceuticals*, **40**(3), 215–18.

Wu, Z. L., Huang, S. L., Ou Yang, D. S. *et al.* (1998). Clomipramine N-demethylation metabolism in human liver microsomes. *Acta Pharmacologica Sinica*, **19**(5), 433–6.

Xu, Z. H., Huang, S. L. & Zhou, H. H. (1996). Inhibition of imipramine N- demethylation by fluvoxamine in Chinese young men. *Acta Pharmacologica Sinica*, **17**(5), 399–402.

Yang, C., Zhao, J. P., Liu, B. *et al.* (2002). Relationships between clozapine steady-state concentration CYP1A2 activity and clinical response in schizophrenic patients. *Journal of Chinese Psychiatry*, **35**(4), 202–5.

Yao, G. Z., Liu, P. & Shu, L. (1997). An open study on efficacy of a new antidepressant citalopram. *Chinese Journal of New Drugs*, **6**(3), 170–3.

Zhang, H. Y. , Shu, L., Li, H. F. *et al.* (2006). Risperidone versus haloperidol in treatment of acute manic episodes of bipolar I disorder: a randomized double-blind controlled multicenter study. *Journal of Chinese Psychiatry*, **39**(1), 33–7.

Zhang, S., Dong, Z. W., Tang, L. *et al.* (2002). Cytochrome P450 2C19 gene polymorphism in four Chinese nationality populations. *Journal of Chinese Medical Genetics*, **19**(1), 52–4.

Zhang, X. B., Sha, W. W., Zhang, Z. J. *et al.* (2005).T102C polymorphism in 5-HT2A receptor gene and tarditive dyskinesia in chronic schizophrenia. *Chinese Mental Health Journal*, **19**(1), 8–10.

Zhao, A. L., Zhao, J. P., Xue, Z. M. *et al.* (2005). Association between polymorphism in the dopamine D4 receptor gene and qualitative and quantitative characters of schizophrenia in Chinese. *Chinese Journal of Psychiatry*, **38**(1), 3–6.

Zhou, M., Liu, P., Zhang, H. Y. *et al.* (2002). Double-blind comparison between risperidone and haloperidol in the treatment of schizophrenic patients. *Chinese Journal of Clinical Pharmacology*, **18**(5), 341–4.

Zhu, B., Xu, Z. H., Wang, W. *et al.* (1999). N-Demethylation of clomipramine in human liver microsomes in vitro. *Journal of Chinese Pharmacology and Toxicology*, **13**(4), 253–9.

# 7

# Variation in psychotropic responses in the Hispanic population

Deborah L. Flores and Ricardo Mendoza

## Introduction

According to the United States Census Bureau (2005), 41.3 million Hispanics reside in the United States and constitute the largest ethnic minority group in the country. Our knowledge base, as it pertains to the nature of the psychopharmacological responsiveness manifested by Hispanics, continues to lag. While the number of psychopharmacological studies including Hispanic patients has increased, they continue to be plagued by the same methodological problems that have been noted in previous reviews (Mendoza & Smith, 2000) and the data is, therefore, difficult to interpret with confidence. To date, the only substantive pharmacogenetic data that has been generated has been in Mexican Americans (a.k.a. Hispanic-Whites), and Hispanics with a Black racial affiliation remain largely ignored. In the following, we review the extant clinical research investigations that have been conducted utilizing Hispanic subjects that have received antidepressant and antipsychotic medications. Pharmacogenetic findings in the Mexican American subgroup are briefly summarized, as is the data regarding drug–diet and drug–herbal interactions. Concluding remarks include a discussion of the limitations and methodological problems associated with this body of research.

## Antidepressants

### Tricyclics

Early landmark studies utilizing Hispanic subjects in the 1980s (Escobar & Tuason, 1980; Marcos & Cancro, 1982) compared the efficacy and response of several tricyclic antidepressants to placebo. They were the first to hint at a possible heightened placebo response in Hispanics and they suggested that certain Hispanic subjects

*Ethno-psychopharmacology: Advances in Current Practice*, eds. C. H. Ng, K.-M. Lin, B. S. Singh and E. Y. K. Chiu. Published by Cambridge University Press. © C. H. Ng, K.-M. Lin, B. S. Singh and E. Y. K. Chiu 2008.

may experience greater side effects at standardized dosages. A later international, multicenter trial comparing the response to fluoxetine or amitriptyline in patients with major depression with anxiety, from five countries (Brazil, n = 52; Colombia, n = 23; Mexico, n = 36; Peru, n = 28; and Venezuela, n = 18) found no differences in efficacy between the two medications other than greater improvement in sleep in the amitriptyline group (Versiani *et al.*, 1999). Twice as many patients (8.8%) receiving amitriptyline dropped out of the study due to side effects when compared to the fluoxetine group (3.9%).

## Selective serotonin re-uptake inhibitors (SSRIs)

An open-label study of paroxetine and fluoxetine (Alonso *et al.*, 1997) in depressed Hispanic (Mexican descent, n = 13) and non-Hispanic females (n = 13) showed no differences in response rates. At variance with the tricyclic data, Hispanic subjects complained of fewer side effects ($2.2 \pm 2.0$ vs. $5.1 \pm 2.5$; $p < 0.005$), but twice as many terminated participation prior to study completion due to non-compliance, intolerable side effects or pregnancy.

Wagner *et al.* (1998) investigated the ethnic differences in antidepressant response to fluoxetine or placebo in 118 depressed, predominantly male, HIV-positive patients (White n = 79, Hispanic n = 17, African American n = 22). Nine Hispanic subjects (53%) dropped out of treatment making the results difficult to interpret. Among completers in the placebo arm, 80% (four out of five) of Hispanic subjects were responders as compared to 36% of African American subjects and 43% of White subjects.

Ferrando *et al.* (1999) conducted an open-label trial of fluoxetine or sertraline in 30 depressed HIV-positive women (including 16 of Puerto Rican or Dominican descent). No differences in treatment response or adverse effects were found between groups.

A small, flexible dose study of citalopram (dosage range = 10–40 mg/day) in 14 Hispanic and 6 non-Hispanic (non-White) depressed HIV-positive patients conducted in Miami also showed no differences in response rate or effective dose between ethnicities (Currier *et al.*, 2004). In addition, Hispanic patients did not have a significantly higher attrition rate compared to non-Hispanics.

Another study with citalopram evaluated its efficacy in the treatment of social anxiety disorder along with co-morbid major depression (Schneier *et al.*, 2003). The outpatients (n = 21) were predominantly Hispanic (76%) and from New York. Response rates for the intent-to-treat sample were 66.7% for social anxiety disorder and 76.2% for major depression. Only one subject was known to have withdrawn secondary to severe side effects. The mean dose of the medication was 37.6 mg/day and there was no placebo control. The depressive symptoms tended to improve faster than the anxious symptoms, consistent with previous reports utilizing SSRIs for the treatment of depression and social anxiety disorder (Stein *et al.*, 2002).

A prospective, randomized, placebo-controlled trial of paroxetine in adults with chronic post-traumatic stress disorder (PTSD) was recently conducted (Marshall *et al.*, 2007). The subjects were New Yorkers, predominantly female (67%) and Hispanic (65.4%). Seventy subjects entered the study and after a one week placebo lead-in, 52 subjects were randomized to placebo or paroxetine for ten weeks. The subjects were treated with a flexible dosage design (mean dosage, 40.4 mg/day). Dropout rates were 32% for paroxetine and 51.9% for placebo. There were no differences in rates of adverse effects between treatment arms. Paroxetine was superior to placebo in ameliorating the primary symptoms of PTSD (56% vs. 22.2%).

An interventional study evaluating the effectiveness of guideline-based care for depression in predominantly low-income minority women (Black, n = 112; "Latinas born in Latin America," n = 134; White, n = 16) was recently reported (Miranda *et al.*, 2003). These women were randomized into treatment with either antidepressants (n = 88) or cognitive behavioral therapy (CBT) (n = 90), or were given a referral to a community mental health clinic (n = 89). Of those receiving antidepressants, 75% continued treatment for at least nine weeks and 45% for at least 24 weeks. Women were initially treated with a flexible dosing of paroxetine (mean dose = 30 mg). Twenty percent of the women on paroxetine were switched to buproprion for either intolerable side effects or lack of response. An adequate course of medication did not differ by ethnicity. No data regarding efficacy of study drug, the emergence of side effects, or ethnicity of the women who required a changed in medication treatment was made available.

A pooled analysis of 14 875 adults (Hispanic, n = 361; White, n = 10 108; African American, n = 547; Asian, n = 112) who participated in 104 double-blind, placebo-controlled paroxetine trials for mood and anxiety disorders was performed to ascertain minority group differences (Roy-Byrne *et al.*, 2005). There were significant differences in rates of response by ethnicity (p = 0.014) with the odds of responding being lower for the Asian and Hispanic subjects compared to the African American and White subjects. There was also a higher placebo response rate in Hispanic subjects. Rapidity of response and emergence of adverse effects were similar across groups.

The results from an open-label, pilot study evaluating the efficacy of fluvoxamine for hypochondriasis were recently published (Fallon *et al.*, 2003). The study sample included six Hispanics (subgroup unknown). Significant improvement (57.1%) was noted for the intent-to-treat group (eight out of fourteen) based on physician-rated and self-rated scales. The sample size was too small to identify differences in response or adverse effects by ethnicity.

### Selective serotonin and norepinephrine re-uptake inhibitors

A large open-label flexible dose study (Sanchez-Lacay *et al.*, 2001) utilizing nefazodone in the treatment of major depression in a predominantly monolingual, Hispanic Caribbean population (Dominican Republic, Puerto Rico, and Cuba) revealed similar response rates and an endpoint mean dosage when compared to previous nefazodone trials with non-Hispanic patients. No serious adverse events were reported, but 42% of the subjects did not complete the study for various reasons including side effects, family, or work responsibilities.

More recently, an analysis of pooled data from seven safety and efficacy trials of duloxetine did not find any differences in efficacy in depressed Hispanics compared with Whites (Lewis-Fernandez *et al.*, 2006). Unfortunately, the sample size for the Hispanic group was very small in comparison to the White cohort (n = 58; White, n = 748), and most likely underpowered to detect any differences. Also, the Hispanic group included Mexicans and Mexican Americans along with Central and South Americans (percentage breakdown is unknown).

## Antipsychotics

It is widely held that differences exist in the usage and dosage of antipsychotics among ethnic minority groups. A number of factors are felt to account for these differences and include sociocultural variables (racial bias, cultural divide between patient and physician, language), as well as biological variables (pharmacogenetic, pharmacokinetic, and pharmacodynamic).

### Racial discrepancies in the use of second-generation antipsychotics (SGAs)

Several studies have indicated minority patients are more likely to be given first-generation antipsychotics (FGAs) such as haloperidol, rather than second-generation antipsychotics (SGAs) such as risperidone or olanzapine (Worrel *et al.*, 2000; Valenstein *et al.*, 2001; Kuno & Rothbard, 2002). Health services researchers have tended to investigate racial discrepancies in SGA use by reviewing large secondary data sets. Copeland *et al.* (2003), examined the National Veterans Administration Pharmacy records for all veterans diagnosed with schizophrenia over a 12-month period in 1999 (n = 69 787). Hispanics comprised 8.5% of the population (Hispanic-White 7.9%, Hispanic-Black 0.6%), African Americans 31%, and white patients 61.3%. Both Hispanics and African Americans had lower odds of receiving an SGA and were much less likely to receive clozapine. Large group discrepancies in the use of these medications (other than clozapine) were not evident. The authors hypothesized this disparity might be linked to the issue of diabetes. Since African Americans and Hispanics are at a greater risk for diabetes compared to Whites, and SGAs such as olanzapine and clozapine have been linked to this illness

(Popli *et al.*, 1997; Henderson, 2002; Sernyak *et al.*, 2002), minority patients may be more hesitant to take these medications compared to White patients. Alternatively, physicians may be less likely to prescribe them in this at-risk population.

Opolka *et al.* (2003) examined Texas Medicaid claims for patients with schizophrenia or schizoaffective disorder during the period of January 1996 to August 1998. These patients had been initiated to treatment with either haloperidol or olanzapine and had no previous use of these medications in the year prior (total, n = 2601; haloperidol, n = 726; olanzapine, n = 1875).

African Americans were about one-third less likely to receive olanzapine compared to White patients in this review. Hispanics, identified as Mexican American, had lower odds of receiving olanzapine in the first ten months of the analysis, but this difference was not significant during the final ten months. The authors explain that the disparity in prescribing patterns between ethnic groups may be due to the psychotic symptomatology manifested by the patients. For example, African Americans with schizophrenia appear to manifest more positive symptoms than other ethnic groups (Lawson, 1986) and traditional antipsychotics, such as haloperidol, are felt to be more effective in treating positive symptoms.

Daumit *et al.* (2003) conducted a series of cross-sectional analyses of outpatient physician visits from 1992–2000 where antipsychotics were prescribed. The data was collected from the National Hospital Ambulatory Medical Care Survey conducted by the National Center for Health Statistics. African Americans had half the odds of receiving an SGA and Hispanics had 40% of the odds, compared with Whites in the early 1990s. During 1998–2000, the frequency of SGA use for nonpsychotic disorders in African Americans was equivalent to Whites but still 25% lower when patients were receiving treatment for a psychotic disorder. The use of SGAs in Hispanics increased and was equal to that of Whites in the late 1990s for all psychiatric diagnoses.

## Efficacy and safety

Utilizing the client database of the Texas Department of Mental Health and Mental Retardation (TMHMR) Patel *et al.* (2006) evaluated the symptom presentation of schizophrenia-spectrum disorders in children and adolescents of different ethnicities (white, n = 30; African American, n = 38; Hispanic, n = 37) and their response to risperidone. Children and adolescents between 6 and 18 years of age with the diagnosis of schizophrenia, schizophreniform, or schizoaffective disorder for whom treatment with risperidone was initiated between January 1995 and June 2000 were eligible for the study. Schizophrenia was the most common diagnosis in the African American (50%) and Hispanic (45%) groups while the White patients were mostly diagnosed with schizoaffective disorder (60%). There were no differences in attrition rates between ethnicities but they were high overall at one year (69%) and two years (93%), and it is possible these patients could have received services outside of the TMHMR system. An analysis of all three ethnic groups showed significant improvement on the Child Behavioral Checklist. There were several limitations to this study. It is unknown if clients received non-pharmacological interventions, and the dosages of risperidone, adherence rates, and use of concomitant medications were not reported.

Early retrospective clinical reviews suggested that US Hispanic and Asian schizophrenic patients were more likely to receive lower doses of antipsychotics compared to White patients (Collazo *et al.*, 1996; Ruiz *et al.*, 1996). They were equally responsive at these lower dosages when compared to Whites and an increased sensitivity to these compounds was hypothesized. A review of the literature yielded only one prospective, double-blind, pilot study comparing the efficacy and side effects of risperidone in Hispanics and a non-Hispanic group (Frackieswisz *et al.*, 2002). Results from the study suggested a faster rate of improvement in the Hispanic patients (n = 10) compared to the non-Hispanic patients (n = 8). A trend towards more extrapyramidal symptoms among Hispanics was also found (p = 0.057). The authors suggested that dosages lower than those typically recommended may be necessary in Hispanic schizophrenics. However, both groups were extremely heterogeneous racially speaking and the samples sizes were exceedingly small.

### Metabolic syndrome, diabetes, and hispanics

An important issue facing all patients, regardless of color, who receive SGAs, particularly olanzapine and clozapine, is the increased incidence of diabetes (American Diabetes Association *et al.*, 2004). Of equal importance, however, is the relationship between SGAs and a condition known as metabolic syndrome. Metabolic syndrome is defined by a cluster of clinical criteria including increased abdominal adiposity, elevated triglycerides with low high-density lipoprotein, hypertension, and impaired fasting glucose or diabetes mellitus (Expert Panel, 2001). This syndrome may be up to three times more prevalent than diabetes among patients with schizophrenia (Meyer *et al.*, 2005) and it poses an increased cardiovascular risk. The third National Health and Nutrition Examination Survey (NHANES III) reported the age-adjusted prevalence of metabolic syndrome in the US population to be 23.7% with a higher prevalence of 32% in Mexican Americans (Ford *et al.*, 2002). A more recent study (Kato *et al.*, 2004) suggested that metabolic syndrome in Hispanics with schizophrenia (predominantly Cuban Americans) was as high as 74% (23 out of 31) compared to 41% (7 out of 17) among non-Hispanics. No definitive association between metabolic syndrome and SGA use was reported. The NIMH funded, Clinical Antipsychotic Trials of Intervention Effective Schizophrenia Trial (CATIE), identified baseline results for the prevalence of metabolic syndrome to be 47.4% (n = 435) among US White patients with schizophrenia and 46.9% (n = 81) among Hispanics. Although both groups were on antipsychotic medications prior to the initiation of this study, there was no reliable documentation of this usage and, as a result, investigators were unable to make reliable causal inferences (Meyer *et al.*, 2005). Furthermore, persons randomized into the CATIE study are unlikely representative of a random sample, and therefore the rates of metabolic syndrome may not accurately reflect those in the community.

## Pharmacogenetics and the Mexican American population

Polymorphic variability in the drug-metabolizing enzymes is an important factor accounting for inter-ethnic and individual differences in drug metabolism. Data regarding the various alleles of CYP2D6, CYP2C19, and CYP2C9 is only available for the Mexican American subgroup.

The CYP2D6 drug-metabolizing enzyme is responsible for the metabolism of many of the drugs that are used in psychiatry and general medicine today. Lam *et al.* (1991) was the first to study the frequency of poor metabolizers (PMs) (4.5%) in a small sample of Mexican Americans (n = 22) in South Texas. Subsequently, Mendoza *et al.* (2001) conducted a study assessing the relationship between CYP2D6 genotype and phenotype in a much larger sample of Mexican Americans in Los Angeles. CYP2D6*2, *3, *4, *5, *10, *17, and gene duplication alleles were examined (n = 349) in relationship to the metabolism of dextromethorphan to dextrophan (n = 285). In that study, a PM frequency of 3.2% was reported and a rapid mean metabolic ratio (MR) of −2.47 among extensive metabolizers (EMs) was identified. A significant gene-dose effect correlated with slow metabolizing mutations. Since a very low frequency of the gene duplication allele was identified, the rapid MR was felt to be due to the relatively low frequency of alleles that have been shown to produce poor or intermediate metabolism among subjects.

In 2005, Casner (2005) conducted a similar study to assess the effects of CYP2D6 polymorphisms in a sample of 75 Mexican Americans from El Paso, Texas. At variance with the Mendoza *et al.* (2001) results, a PM frequency of 6% was reported. The study sample also manifested a rapid mean MR of −2.54 among EMs. The frequency of the *4 allele was 0.17 in the El Paso subjects and was significantly higher than in the Los Angeles sample (0.11). The increased presence of the *4 mutation accounted for the higher PM frequency in El Paso subjects. Differences in sample size, Mexican ancestry qualifiers, and historical immigration patterns into the United States were hypothesized to explain the differences between the El Paso and Los Angeles study samples.

Two additional pharmacogenetic studies utilized the Los Angeles Mexican American study sample previously cited (Mendoza *et al.*, 2001). First, Luo *et al.* (2005) extended the CYP2D6 genotyping analysis further to include *6, *7, *8,

\*9, \*11,\*14, \*29, \*41, \*45, and \*46 alleles. These results, taken together with the results from the Mendoza *et al.* (2001) study, show that the \*4, \*5, and \*6 null alleles, along with the reduced functional alleles \*9, \*10, and \*41 are the major cause of reduced dextromethorphan metabolism in Mexican Americans. Subsequently, Luo *et al.* (2006) performed the first analysis of the CYP2C19 polymorphism in Mexican Americans. Their results showed the frequency of phenotype PM or PM based on CYP2C19 genotype is low in Mexican Americans when compared with results from other ethnic minority groups (African Americans, East Asians, Southeast Asians, Caucasians, $p \leq 0.035$). In a similar fashion to the CYP2D6 findings, Mexican Americans had a very low frequency of CYP2C19 null allele, which was felt to account for the low PM frequency.

Lastly, Llerena *et al.* (2004) compared the CYP2C9 polymorphisms \*1,\*2,\*3,\*4,\*5, and \*6 in Mexican Americans (n = 98) and Spanish subjects (n = 102). Lower frequencies of the variant CYP2C9\*2, one of two alleles reported to have altered catalytic activity, were found among the Mexican Americans. Since no phenotypic comparisons were conducted in this study, the clinical implications remain unclear. The authors suggest the need for further studies to assess whether the drug metabolism of medications such as warfarin may be affected in this population.

## Drug–diet and drug–herbal interactions

Hispanics are more likely to use herbal therapies because they believe they are less costly, more efficacious, and have fewer side effects than conventional medications (Gupchup *et al.*, 2006). Ng *et al.* (2006) attempted to better document the use of herbal therapies in minorities by examining the charts from 453 psychiatric outpatients in Southern California (48% Hispanic). Insomnia (37%) and stress (29%) were the most commonly cited reasons for taking herbal remedies and the most frequent herbals reported were ingested as teas – chamomile (*manzanilla*) and "*siete azahares*," or "seven blossoms." *Siete azahares* is believed to have antidepressant and anxiolytic effects similar to benzodiazepines (Santos *et al.*, 1994; Beaubrun & Gray, 2000). This may be due in part to one of its ingredients, *Valeriana officinalis* (valerian), which is also used independently in the treatment of insomnia. Valerian is a sedative, which improves sleep quality and shortens sleep latency. It is commonly used in the Hispanic community (Schulz *et al.*, 2001; Mischoulon, 2002; Dominguez *et al.*, 2000). There are no reports of herbal–drug interactions with the above-mentioned herbal therapies, but there have been some rare adverse reactions linked to valerian including vision blurriness, hepatotoxicity, and dystonias (Schulz *et al.*, 2001). There may also be a carcinogenic risk with the use of valerian imported from Mexico (Schulz *et al.*, 2001).

In a recent retrospective review of the medical records of diabetic Hispanic women (n = 81), Johnson *et al.* (2006) reported that 15.4% of these records documented the use of herbal treatments, which included, among others, *Piper methysticum* (Kava Kava) and *Hypericum perforatum* (St. John's Wort). These represent the most well studied herbal therapies used for psychiatric disorders, but heretofore not felt to be commonly used in the Hispanic community. Kava is known to have anxiolytic effects and has been evaluated in the treatment of generalized anxiety disorder (Watkins *et al.*, 2001; Conner & Davidson, 2002). It has been associated with hepatoxicity (Campo *et al.*, 2002) and a case report suggested possible additive effects with benzodiazepines resulting in a coma-like state (Almeida & Grimsley, 1996). St. John's Wort was once believed to be effective for mild depression (Schrader, 2000), though a more recent study tempers this conclusion (Lecrubier *et al.*, 2002). It is an inducer of CYP3A4 and therefore decreases the serum levels of several medications including cyclosporine, oral contraceptives, warfarin, digoxin, and theophylline (Izzo & Ernst, 2001). It is also a mild monoamine oxidase inhibitor and may precipitate a mild serotonin syndrome if given with SSRIs (Fugh-Berman, 2000).

While CYP2D6 and CYP2C19 are felt to be primarily under genetic control, CYP1A2 and CYP3A4 are felt to be highly influenced by environmental and dietary factors and therefore susceptible to inhibition or induction (Mendoza & Smith, 2000). Heavy smoking, charcoal cooking, and air pollution are associated with the induction of CYP1A2 (Conney *et al.*, 1977) and dosages of certain medications such as olanzapine, fluxoamine, and amitriptyline may need to be lowered because their serum levels may increase in the face of these factors. The enzyme CYP3A4 metabolizes many psychotropic drugs including benzodiazepines (alprazolam, diazepam, midazolam), buspirone, nefazadone, and haloperidol. The intestinal form of this enzyme is inhibited by flavonoids such as quercetin, kaempferol, and naringenin (Fukuda *et al.*, 1997). Quercetin, which is strongly inhibitory, is found in grapefruit juice and corn (Fukuda *et al.*, 1997; Palma-Aguirre *et al.*, 1994). It is well known that corn is a dietary staple in Hispanic cultures, regardless of race. The serum levels of drugs metabolized by CYP3A4 may be higher in patients who eat large amounts of corn producing an artificial hypersensitivity.

## Conclusions

The research literature regarding the pharmacological treatment of Hispanics is sorely lacking and suffers from a number of methodological problems. To begin with, we must do a better job of clearly defining the Hispanic population. Official census bureau tracking of this ethnic minority group now includes the additional qualifier of race. Future research with Hispanic subjects should incorporate the

Census Bureau taxonomy. This standardization would eliminate ambiguities and allow for a better interpretation of results.

Second, while we applaud the fact that more Hispanics are being included in clinical studies, the sample sizes continue to be small, limiting the interpretations that can be made from the data. In some cases, multiple studies have been pooled together to increase the "Hispanic" sample size. This is methodologically less rigorous as there may be variability in the methods employed between studies, for example inter-rater differences.

Third, many pharmacological studies focusing on Hispanics are methodologically flawed. Many have open-label designs, others are retrospective reviews of medical records or post-hoc analyses assessing for ethnic differences in drug response. Studies employing these research designs are much less conclusive than prospective, blinded, and placebo-controlled investigations. Only one prospective study of antipsychotic efficacy including Hispanics was revealed in our literature search and that only included eight subjects. Other efficacy studies have analyzed large data sets to examine for racial differences. Secondary data sets are limited by a number of constraints and caution must be exercised when making causal inferences from these data. Very few studies have the a-priori hypothesis that ethnicity might affect efficacy or side effects, and therefore are not designed to maximize the ability to detect such differences. Also, while the major pharmaceutical companies should be praised for their recent efforts to include ethnic minority groups into their phase III and post-marketing clinical trials, these companies have recently come under scrutiny owing to possible data manipulation, either consciously or inadvertently. Caution should be exercised when reading the results from industry-sponsored clinical trials.

Fourth, proper assessment of level of acculturation is missing from most drug studies that enroll Hispanic subjects. Cultural beliefs and explanatory models are known to shape adherence rates and possibly placebo response. There is often no mention of immigrant status or language preference and proficiency of the subjects studied. Practically speaking, most studies exclude monolingual Spanish speakers. If they are included, it is important to assess whether psychiatric instruments being used for assessment have been translated into Spanish and properly validated. These issues are important in order to safeguard the accuracy of diagnosis, which is the cornerstone of proper pharmacological management.

Fifth, the increased risk of obesity and diabetes mellitus in Hispanics warrants careful consideration of SGA use in this population. Although there is variance in the data from studies assessing the incidence of metabolic syndrome in Hispanics being administered SGAs, one study pointed to a significantly higher incidence compared to non-Hispanics. Further research in this area is warranted.

Finally, pharmacogenetic data regarding the drug-metabolizing enzymes continues to be available only for the Mexican American population. The results from these pharmacogenetic studies accurately reflect the unique genetic admixture in Mexican Americans, which is largely influenced by ancestral Amerindian settlers of the Americas and conquering Eastern European Spaniards. These data show a low frequency of PMs and indicate little need for dosage adjustments in this Hispanic subgroup. This evidence notwithstanding, dietary influencers in the form of corn, grapefruit juice, and charcoal grilling, along with possible effects from herbal remedies used by this minority group must be taken into consideration in order to better individualize pharmacological interventions. Future large-scale studies of CYP2D6 and CYP2C19 examining the relationship between genotyping and phenotyping in Hispanics with a Black affiliation must be undertaken to assess for unique polymorphic variability in these subgroups.

## REFERENCES

Almeida, J. C. & Grimsley, E. W. (1996). Coma from the health food store: interaction between kava and alprazolam. *Ann. Intern. Med.*, **125**, 940–1.

Alonso, M., Val, E. & Rapaport, M. H. (1997). An open-label study of SSRI treatment in depressed Hispanic and non-Hispanic women. *J. Clin. Psychiatry*, **58**, 31.

American Diabetes Association, American Psychiatrics Association, American Association of Clinical Endocrinologists, North American Association for the Study of Obesity (2004). Consensus development conference on antipsychotic drugs and obesity and diabetes. *J. Clin. Psychiatry*, **65**, 267–72.

Beaubrun, G. & Gray, G. E. (2000). A review of herbal medicines for psychiatric disorders. *Psychiatr. Serv.*, **51**, 1130–4.

Campo, J. V., McNabb, J., Perel, J. M. *et al.* (2002). Kava-induced fulminant hepatic failure. *J. Am. Acad. Child Adoles. Psychiatr.*, **41**, 631–2.

Collazo, J., Tam, R., Sramek, J. J. & Herrera, J. (1996). Neuroleptic dosing in Hispanic and Asian inpatients with schizophrenia. *Mt. Sinai. J. Med.*, **63**, 285–90.

Conner, K. M. & Davidson, J. R. (2002). A placebo-controlled study of kava kava in generalized anxiety disorder. *Int. Clin. Psychopharmacol.*, **17**, 185–8.

Conney, A. H., Pantuck, E. J., Hsiao, K. C. *et al.* (1977). Regulation of drug metabolism in man by environmental chemical and diet. *Federation Proceedings*, **36**, 1647–52.

Copeland, L. A., Zeber, J. E., Valenstein, M. & Blow, F. C. (2003). Racial disparity in the use of atypical antipsychotic medications among veterans. *Am. J. Psychiatry*, **160**, 1817–22.

Casner, P. (2005). The effect of CYP2D6 polymorphisms on dextromethorphan metabolism in Mexican Americans. *J. Clin. Pharmacol.*, **45**, 1230–5.

Currier, M. B., Molina, G. & Kato, M. (2004). Citalopram treatment of major depressive disorder in Hispanic HIV and AIDS patients: a prospective study. *Psychosomatics*, **45**, 210–16.

Daumit, G. L., Crum, R. M., Guallar, E., Powe, N. R. *et al.* (2003). Outpatient prescriptions for atypical antispsychotics for African Americans, Hispanics, and whites in the United States. *Arch. Gen. Psychiatry*, **60**, 121–8.

Dominguez, R. A., Bravo-Valverde, R. L., Kaplowitz, B. R. & Cott, J. M. (2000). Valerian as a hypnotic for Hispanic patients. *Cultur. Divers. Ethnic Minor. Psychol.*, **6**, 84–92.

Escobar, J. I. & Tuason, V. B. (1980). Antidepressant agents – a cross-cultural study. *Psychopharmacol. Bull.*, **16**, 49–52.

Expert Panel on Detection, Evaluation and Treatment of High Blood Cholesterol in Adults (2001). Executive summary of the third report of the National Cholesterol Education Program (NCEP) expert panel on detection, evaluation, and treatment of high blood cholesterol in adults (adult treatment panel III). *JAMA*, **285**, 2486–97.

Fallon, B. A., Qureshi, A. I., Schneier, F., Sanchez-Lacy, A. *et al.* (2003). An open trial of fluvoxamine for hypochondriasis. *Psychosomatics*, **44**, 298–303.

Ferrando, S. J., Rabkin, J. G., Moore, G. M. & Rabkin, R. (1999). Antidepressant treatment of depression in HIV-seropositive women. *J. Clin. Psychiatry*, **60**, 741–6.

Ford, E. S., Giles, W. H. & Dietz, W. H. (2002). Prevalence of metabolic syndrome among US adults: findings from the third national health and nutrition examination survey. *JAMA*, **287**, 356–9.

Frackiesicz, E. J., Herrera, J. M., Sramek, J. J., Collazo, J. *et al.* (2002). Risperidone in the treatment of Hispanic inpatients with schizophrenia: a pilot study. *Psychiatry*, **65**, 317–74.

Fugh-Berman, A. (2000). Herb–drug interactions. *Lancet*, **355**, 134–8.

Fukuda, K., Ohra, T. & Yamazoe, Y. (1997). Grapefruit component interacting with rat and human P450 CYP3A: possible involvement on non-flavonoid components in drug interaction. *Biol. Pharm. Bull.*, **20**, 560–4.

Gupchup, G. V., Abhyankar, U. L., Worley, M. M., Raisch, D. W. *et al.* (2006). Relationships between Hispanic ethnicity and attitudes and beliefs toward herbal medicine in older adults. *Res. Social Adm. Pharm.*, **2**, 266–79.

Henderson, D. C. (2002). Atypical antipsychotic-induced diabetes mellitus: how strong is the evidence? *CNS Drugs*, **16**, 77–89.

Izzo, A. A. & Ernst, E. (2001). Interactions between herbal medicines and prescribed drugs: a systematic review. *Drugs*, **61**, 2163–75.

Johnson, L., Strich, H., Taylor, A., Timmermann, B. *et al.* (2006). Use of herbal remedies by diabetic Hispanic women in the southwestern united states. *Phytother. Res.*, **20**, 250–5.

Kato, M. M., Currier, M. B., Gomez, C. M. *et al.* (2004). Prevalence of metabolic syndrome in Hispanic and non-Hispanic patients with schizophrenia. *Prim. Care Companion J. Clin. Psychiatry*, **6**, 74–7.

Kuno, E. & Rothbard, A. B. (2002). Racial disparities in antipsychotic prescription patterns for patients with schizophrenia. *Am. J. Psychiatry*, **159**, 567–72.

Lam, Y. E. F., Castro, D. T. & Dunn, J. F. (1991). Drug metabolizing capacity in Mexican Americans. *Clin. Pharmacol. Ther.*, **49**, 159.

Lawson, W. B. (1986). Clinical issues in pharmacotherapy of African Americans. *Psychopharmacol. Bull.*, **32**, 275–81.

Lecrubier, Y., Clerc, G., Didi, R. & Kieser, M. (2002). Efficacy of St. John's Wort extract WS 5570 in major depression: a double-blind, placebo-controlled trial. *Am. J. Psychiatry*, **159**, 1361–6.

Lewis-Fernandez, R., Blanco, C., Mallinkcrodt, C. H., Wohlreich, M. M. *et al.* (2006). Duloxetine in the treatment of major depressive disorder: comparisons of safety and efficacy in US Hispanic and majority Caucasian patients. *J. Clin. Psychiatry*, **67**, 1379–90.

LLerena, A., Dorado, P., O'Kirwan, F. *et al.* (2004). Lower frequency of CYP2C9 *2 in Mexican-Americans compared to Spaniards. *Pharmacogenomics J.*, **4**, 403–6.

Luo, H. R., Gaedigk, A, Aloumanis, V. & Wan, Y. Y. (2005). Identification of CYP2D6 impaired functional alleles in Mexican Americans. *Eur. J. Clin. Pharmacol.*, **61**, 797–802.

Luo, H. R., Poland, R., Lin, K. M. & Wan, Y. Y. (2006). Genetic polymorphism of cytochrome P450 2C19 in Mexican Americans a cross ethnic comparative study. *Clin. Pharmacol. Ther.*, **80**, 33–40.

Marcos, L. R. & Cancro, R. (1982). Pharmacotherapy of Hispanic depressed patients: clinical observations. *Am. J. Psychother.*, **36**, 505–12.

Marshall, R. D., Lewis-Fernandez, R., Blanco, C., Simpson, H. B. *et al.* (2007). A controlled trial of paroxetine for chronic PTSD, dissociation, and interpersonal problems in mostly minority adults. *Depress. Anxiety*, **24**, 77–84.

Mendoza, R. & Smith, M. (2000). The Hispanic response to psychotropic medications. In P. Ruiz, ed., *Ethnicity and Psychopharmacology*. (Review of Psychiatry Series, Vol. 19, No. 4; J. O. Oldham and M. B. Riba series eds.) Washington, DC: American Psychiatric Press, pp. 55–89.

Mendoza, R., Wan, Y. J., Poland, R. E. *et al.* (2001). CYP 2D6 in a Mexican American population. *Clin. Pharmacol. Ther.,* **70**, 552–60.

Meyer, J. M., Nasrallah, H. A., McEvoy, J. P., Goff, D. C. *et al.* (2005). The clinical antipsychotic trials of intervention effectiveness trial: clinical comparison of subgroups with and without metabolic syndrome. *Schizophr. Res.*, **80**, 9–18.

Miranda, J., Chung, J. Y., Green, B. L., Krupnick, J. *et al.* (2003). Treating depression in predominantly low-income young minority women. *JAMA*, **290**, 57–65.

Mischoulon, D. (2002). The herbal anxiolytics kava and valerian for anxiety and insomnia. *Psychiatric Annals*, **32**, 55–60.

Ng, B., Camacho, A., Simmons, A. & Matthews, S. C. (2006). Ethnicity and use of alternative products in psychiatric patients. *Psychosomatics*, **47**, 408–13.

Opolka, J. L., Rascati, K. L., Brown, C. M., Barner, J. C. *et al.* (2003). Ethnic differences in use of antipsychotic medication among Texas Medicaid clients with schizophrenia. *J. Clin. Psychiatry*, **64**, 635–9.

Palma-Aguirre, J. A., Nava-Rangel, J., Hoyo-Vadillo, C. *et al.* (1994). Influence of Mexican diet on nifedipine pharmacodynamics in healthy volunteers. *Proc. West. Pharmacol. Soc.*, **37**, 85–6.

Patel, N. C., Crismon, M. L., Shafer, A., De Leon, A., Lopez, M. *et al.* (2006). Ethnic variation in symptoms and response to risperidone in youths with schizophrenia-spectrum disorders. *Soc. Psychiatry. Psychiatr. Epidemiol.*, **41**, 341–6.

Popli, A. P., Konicki, P. E., Jurjus, G. J., Fuller, M. A. *et al.* (1997). Clozapine and associated diabetes mellitus. *J. Clin. Psychiatry*, **58**, 108–11.

Roy-Byrne, P. P., Philip, P., Pitts, C. & Christi, J. (2005). Paroxetine response and tolerability among ethnic minority patients with mood or anxiety disorders: a pooled analysis. *J. Clin. Psychiatry*, **66**, 1228–33.

Ruiz, S., Chu, P., Sramek, J. J. & Herrera, J. (1996). Neuroleptic dosing in Asians and Hispanic outpatients with schizophrenia. *Mt. Sinai J. Med.*, **63**, 306–9.

Sanchez-Lacay, J. A., Lewis-Fernandez, R., Goetz, D., Blanco, C. *et al.* (2001). Open trial of nefazodone among Hispanics with major depression: efficacy, tolerability, and adherence issues. *Depress. Anxiety*, **13**, 118–24.

Santos, M. S., Ferreira, F., Faro, C. *et al.* (1994). The amount of GABA present in aqueous extracts of valerian is sufficient to account for [3H] GABA release in synaptosomes. *Planta Med.*, **60**, 475–6.

Schneier, F. R., Blanco, C., Campeas, R., Lewis-Fernandez, R. *et al.* (2003). Citalopram treatment of social anxiety disorder with comorbid major depression. *Depress. Anxiety*, **17**, 191–6.

Schrader, E. (2000). Equivalence of St John's Wort extract (Ze 117) and fluoxetine: a randomized, controlled study in mild–moderate depression. *Int. Clin. Psychopharmacol.*, **15**, 61–8.

Schulz, V., Hansel, R. & Tyler, V. E. (2001). *Rational Phytotherapy: A Physicians' Guide to Herbal Medicine*, 4th ed. Berlin: Springer.

Sernyak, M. J., Leslie, D. L., Alarcon, R. D., Losonczy, M. F. *et al.* (2002). Association of diabetes mellitus with use of atypical neuroleptics in the treatment of schizophrenia. *Am. J. Psychiatry*, **159**, 561–6.

Stein, D. J., Stein, M. B., Pitts, C. D., Kumar, R. *et al.* (2002). Predictors of response to pharmacotherapy in social anxiety disorder: an analysis of three placebo-controlled paroxetine trials. *J. Clin. Psychiatry*, **63**, 152–5.

Wagner, G. J., Mague, S. & Rabkin, J. G. (1998). Ethnic differences in response to fluoxetine in a controlled trial with depressed HIV-positive patients. *Psychiatr. Serv.*, **9**, 239–40.

Watkins, L. L., Conner, K. M. & Davidson, J. R. (2001). Effect of kava extract on vagal cardiac control in generalized anxiety disorder; preliminary findings. *J. Psychopharmacol.*, **15**, 283–6.

Worrel, J. A., Marken, P. A., Beckman, S. E. *et al.* (2000). Atypical antipsychotic agents: a critical review. *Am. J. Health Syst. Pharm.*, **57**, 238–58.

US Census Bureau News (2005) Hispanic population passes 40 million. Washington, DC: US Census Bureau, June 9, 2005.

Valenstein, M., Copeland, L. A., Owen, R., Blow, F. C. *et al.* (2001). Adherence assessments and the use of depot antipsychotic medications in patients with schizophrenia. *J. Clin. Psychiatry*, **62**, 545–54.

Versiani, M., Ontiveros, A., Mazzotti, G., Ospina, J. *et al.* (1999). Fluoxetine versus amitriptyline in the treatment of major depression with associated anxiety (anxious depression): a double-blind comparison. *Int. Clin. Psychopharmacol.*, **14**, 321–7.

# 8

# Identifying inter-ethnic variations in psychotropic response in African Americans and other ethnic minorities

William B. Lawson

## Introduction

The United States is becoming more diverse, ethnically and culturally. This process is happening primarily through immigration and also to some extent from differential birth rates of various ethnic groups. Over a third of today's Americans are considered ethnic minorities. Currently Hispanics and African Americans each make up about 15% of the population. It is anticipated that individuals of European ancestry will become less than a majority in 2050 (US Census, 2000).

These population changes have important implications for pharmacotherapy. It is now widely accepted that genetic differences between the various ethnic groups are quite small and probably less than individual differences. The recent experience with the newly approved congestive heart failure medication, BiDil, suggests that even minor differences can have significant pharmacological consequences.

The concept for BiDil developed from studies conducted in veterans administration hospitals on the effectiveness of the combination of two older drugs, hydralazine and isosorbide dinitrate, on congestive heart failure. Neither drug had an indication for congestive heart failure. No significant effect was seen in these studies on the general veteran population with congestive heart failure. However, a post-hoc analysis showed that the combination agents were effective for the African Americans in the study (Carson et al., 1999). A subsequent larger study, the African American Heart Failure Trial confirmed the efficacy of the combination medication in a patient population with congestive heart failure that was exclusively African American (Taylor et al., 2004). Presumably its effectiveness in African Americans may be related to diminished bioavailability of nitrous oxide in African Americans, although the actual mechanism has not been established.

*Ethno-psychopharmacology: Advances in Current Practice*, eds. C. H. Ng, K.-M. Lin, B. S. Singh and E. Y. K. Chiu. Published by Cambridge University Press. © C. H. Ng, K.-M. Lin, B. S. Singh and E. Y. K. Chiu 2008.

Subsequently the medication was approved for self identified African Americans by the Federal Drug Administration (FDA), the first time a medication was approved for a specific racial group (US Food and Drug Administration, 2005). This combination was then marketed as BiDil. The approval led to a great deal of controversy and discussion, much of it critical, about the FDA decision. The findings from these trials, however, provide evidence that ethnicity can make a difference in clinical treatment response (Sankar & Kahn, 2005).

These findings also highlighted the importance of the disparity in participation of African Americans and ethnic minorities in clinical trials. The Surgeon General's Supplemental Report on Mental Health reviewed minority participation in clinical trials and noted that participation was very small compared to Whites of European ancestry (US Department of Health and Human Services, 2001). No single ethnic group exceeded 10% participation. Such small numbers meant that there was not sufficient power in most studies to analyze treatment efficacy for any ethnic minority group. We surveyed all biological psychiatry studies done during the 1980s and found similar results. Ethnicity was rarely identified, and when it was African Americans represented no more then 6% of the subjects (Lawson, 1990).

## Biological factors and clinical implications

Research in psychopharmacology has shown that ethnicity must be considered in psychiatry as well (Lawson, 1986; Pi & Simpson, 2005). Early clinical trials with antipsychotic and antidepressant medications showed that ethnic minorities may respond when given the same doses as Caucasians, and may have more side effects (Lawson, 1986; Lawson, 1990). However, dosing cannot be used as a measure of appropriate pharmacotherapy because an extensive literature has shown that African Americans often receive higher doses of antipsychotics despite evidence of more side effects.

Excessive dosing appears to be a consequence of the therapist's attitude to the patient rather then clinical response. Higher medication doses appear to be the result of a lack of therapist involvement with the patient (Segal et al., 1996). We reported that African American patients diagnosed with schizophrenia were perceived as being more violent by the staff even when they were less violent then Caucasians in the same setting based on objective information (Lawson, 1986; Lawson et al., 1984). This excessive dosing may explain in part the doubling of the risk for the persistent movement disorder tardive dyskinesia in African Americans (Morgenstern & Glazer, 1993; Jeste et al., 1995; Glazer et al., 1994; Lindamer et al., 1999)

Biological factors that may influence pharmacological response and side effects include pharmacokinetics such as protein binding, distribution, metabolism, or excretion. They may also include pharmacodynamics such as receptor or tissue sensitivity (Pi & Simpson, 2005). Recent research, however, has focused on the cytochrome P (CYP) system. Over 90% of drugs in clinical use are metabolized by the CYP450 family of liver isoenzymes (Bradford, 2002). These drugs would include the antipsychotic and antidepressant medications in common use. This enzyme may show reduced, "normal" activity, or enhanced activity leading to decreased or increased drug metabolism, and increased or reduced plasma concentrations of a medication that may have clinical consequences (Lin, 2001). While CYP2D6 accounts for less than 2% of total CYP450 liver enzymes, it accounts for 25% of the metabolism of drugs in common use (Bradford, 2002). Recent studies have shown that individuals with deficient CYP2D6 alleles are more likely to have extrapyramidal side effects on antipsychotics and to discontinue treatment (Chillevoort *et al.*, 2002; de Leon *et al.*, 2005).

Ethnic differences in CYP2D6 have been more thoroughly documented than with the other isoenzyme (Bradford, 2002). Over 70% of Caucasians but only about half of Asians, Sub-Saharan Africans, and African Americans have fully functional CYP2D6 alleles – alleles that code for "normal" metabolic activity. Approximately 50% of Asian and people of African ancestry have reduced function or nonfunctioning alleles. As a consequence, many older psychotropic medications are metabolized more slowly and plasma levels would be higher. Thus individuals of African and Asian ancestry would have an increased risk of side effects and should receive lower dose for a therapeutic response when compared to Caucasians of European descent (Lin, 2001; Lawson, 2000).

Newer antipsychotic agents may not be as extensively metabolized through the CYP2D6 system. A multisite randomized control trial compared haloperidol, a first-generation antipsychotic agent metabolized through CYP2D6, with olanzanpine, a second-generation agent metabolized through CYP1A2 and with CYP2D6 a minor pathway. More drug-induced movement disorder was seen with haloperidol (Tollefson *et al.*, 1997). Post-hoc analysis by race found fewer reports of extrapyramidal symptoms and dyskinesia (4%) with olanzapine in patients of African descent, than with haloperidol (22%) (Tran *et al.*, 1999). In addition we found ethnic variation in the risk for movement disorders between those of African, Asian, and European Caucasian ancestry for haloperidol. No such variation was seen for olanzapine. While newer antipsychotic agents may reduce the risk for drug-induced movement disorder for ethnic minorities, it, however, may come at the price of increased risk for obesity, diabetes, and the metabolic syndrome (Bailey, 2003; Fenton & Chavez, 2006).

Lithium presents yet another model of ethnic variation in side effects and response. It is well established that African Americans show a higher red blood cell (RBC) to plasma ratio of lithium concentration when compared to Asians and

Caucasians (Okpaku *et al.*, 2005; Strickland *et al.*, 1995). Presumably this difference is a result of the tendency of African Americans to retain sodium. Sodium retention offered a selective survival advantage for slaves bought to America over the middle passage since hyponatremia was believed the major cause of mortality (Hildreth & Saunders, 1991).

The clinical significance of this ethnic difference for psychiatry was found later. A study examining lithium tolerability found more side effects in African American patients with high RBC/plasma ratio even when the lithium levels were in the therapeutic range (Strickland *et al.*, 1995). It is not known whether African Americans require lower doses and will respond with lower plasma levels. We do know that African Americans with mood disorders are less likely to be prescribed lithium either as primary treatment or adjunctive therapy (Valenstein *et al.*, 2006; Kilbourne & Pincus, 2006). It is unknown as to whether the lack of tolerability at usual therapeutic doses is a factor.

A recent study showed yet another mechanism for ethnic differences in pharmacological response. The STAR*D study was a prospective study of the effectiveness of the newest generation of antidepressants (Trivedi *et al.*, 2006). Patients were genotyped to find genetic predictors of treatment response to the selective serotonin re-uptake inhibitor (SSRI), citalopram. A relationship was found between the HTR2A gene, which codes for the serotonin 2A receptor, and treatment response (McMahon *et al.*, 2006). The allele is six times more frequent in Whites than in African Americans and in fact African Americans were less responsive to citalopram. It is unknown whether these findings can be generalized to other SSRIs. It is significant that African Americans with depression are less likely to be treated with SSRIs (Melfi *et al.*, 2000).

## Research participation

These findings emphasize the importance of including ethnic minorities in clinical trials in sufficient numbers and to do intra-ethnic analysis. Failure to do so will mean that guidelines for new pharmacological products will be relevant mostly to treating Caucasians only. Ethnic minorities are left at risk for possible idiosyncratic side effects, inappropriate dosing, or lack of efficacy.

The argument is often made that African Americans and other ethnic minorities do not participate in clinical trials because they do not want to. African Americans in particular were thought to be suspicious of participation because of previous experiences of exploitation and manhandling of vulnerable minority groups (Melfi *et al.*, 2000; Corbie-Smith *et al.*, 1999). The Tusgekee syphilis study is often cited as a reason for mistrust (Shavers *et al.*, 2000; Shavers *et al.*, 2002; Corbie-Smith *et al.*, 1999). This study was a federally funded study of the long-term consequences of syphilis on African American men initially started before antibiotics were available.

However, the participants were not given treatment when they became available and were not informed that they were not given optimal treatment. African Americans aware of this study are less likely to participate in research (Shavers *et al.*, 2000; Hamilton *et al.*, 2006). Even African Americans unaware of the study often mistrust research that might involve physically intrusive methods (Hamilton *et al.*, 2006). This mistrust applies to psychiatric research as well (Wendler *et al.*, 2006).

Recent findings have challenged the view that lack of participation is a result of African American attitudes about research. The consent rate by race and ethnicity was examined in all the published health research studies done in the United States, Western Europe, and Australia (Wendler *et al.*, 2006). No significant racial or ethnic differences were seen even when the US alone was studied. This report found no significant difference between ethnicities, with all groups showing above 80% consent rates. For clinical intervention studies African Americans had a non-significantly higher and Hispanics a significantly higher consent rate than non-Hispanic Whites.

The African-American Heart Failure Trial showed that a large number of African Americans can be recruited in sufficient numbers with enough power to show efficacy in a clinical trial. In psychiatry the large STAR*D study of depression was made up of 24% minorities (Trivedi *et al.*, 2006). The recently completed Clinical Antipsychotic Trials of Intervention Effectiveness (CATIE) was able to recruit enough African Americans to make up about one third of its participants (Stroup *et al.*, 2006).

## Conclusion

In an increasingly multiethnic nation, pharmacological and genetic research is showing that ethnicity must be considered in the development of new treatments for psychiatric disorders. Small efficacy studies and large effectiveness studies are showing the value of addressing inter-ethnic variation in pharmacotherapy. Participation by ethnic minorities in clinical trials continues to be low not because of participant attitudes but because of a failure to target minority populations. Large-scale effectiveness studies in psychiatry have shown both the importance and the practicality of adequate recruitment of minorities.

## REFERENCES

Bailey, R. K. (2003). Atypical psychotropic medications and their adverse effects: a review for the African-American primary care physician. *J. Natl. Med. Assoc.*, **95**, 37–44.

Bradford, L. D. (2002). CYP2D6 allele frequency in European Caucasians, Asians, Africans and their descendants. *Pharmacogenomics*, **3**, 229–43.

Carson, P., Ziesche, S., Johnson, G. *et al.* (1999). Racial differences in response to therapy for heart failure: analysis of the vasodilator-heart failure trials. *J. Card. Fail.*, **5**, 178–87.

Corbie-Smith, G., Thomas, S. B., Williams, M. V. *et al.* (1999). Attitudes and beliefs of African-Americans toward participation in medical research. *J. Gen. Int. Med.*, **14**, 537–46.

de Leon, J., Susce, M. T., Pan, R. M., Fairchild, M. *et al.* (2005). The CYP2D6 poor metabolizer phenotype may be associated with risperidone adverse drug reactions and discontinuation. *J. Clin. Psychiatry*, **66**, 15–27.

Fenton, W. S. & Chavez, M. R. (2006). Medication-induced weight gain and dyslipidemia in patients with schizophrenia. *Am. J. Psychiatry*, **163**, 1697–704.

Glazer, W. M., Morgenstern, H. & Doucette, J. (1994). Race and tardive dyskinesia among outpatients at a CMHC. *Hosp. Comm. Psychiatry*, **45**, 38–42.

Hamilton, L. A., Aliyu, M. H., Lyons, P.D . *et al.* (2006). African-American community attitudes and perceptions toward schizophrenia and medical research: an exploratory study. *J. Natl. Med. Assoc.*, **98**, 18–27.

Hildreth, C. & Saunders, O. (1991). Hypertension in Blacks: clinical overview. *Cardiovascular Clin.*, **21**, 85–96.

Jeste, D. V., Caligiuri, M. P. & Paulsen, J. S. (1995). Risk of tardive dyskinesia in older patients: a prospective longitudinal study of 266 patients. *Arch. Gen. Psychiatry*, **52**, 756–65.

Kilbourne, A. M. & Pincus, H. A. (2006). Patterns of psychotropic medication use by race among veterans with bipolar disorder. *Psychiatry Serv.*, **57**, 123–6.

Lawson, W. B. (1986). Racial and ethnic factors in psychiatric research. *Hosp. Comm. Psychiatry*, **37**, 50–4.

Lawson, W. B. (1990). Biological markers in neuropsychiatric disorders: racial and ethnic factors. In E. Sorel, ed., *Family, Culture, and Psychobiology*. New York: Levas.

Lawson, W. B. (2000). Issues in the pharmacotherapy of African American. In P. Ruiz, ed., *Review of Psychiatry*. Washington DC: American Association Press, Vol. 19(4), pp. 37–53.

Lawson, W. B., Yesavage, J. A. & Werner, R. D. (1984). Race, violence, and psychopathology. *J. Clin. Psychiatry*, **45**, 294–7.

Lin, K. M. (2001). Biological differences in depression and anxiety across races and ethnic groups. *J. Clin. Psychiatry*, **62**(13), 13–19.

Lindamer, L., Lacro, J. P. & Jeste, D.V. (1999). Relationship of ethnicity to the effects of antipsychotic medication. In J. M. Herrara, W. B. Lawson and J. J. Sramek, eds., *Cross Cultural Psychiatry*. Sussex: John Wiley & Sons.

McMahon, F. J., Buervenich, S., Charney, D. *et al.* (2006). Variation in the gene encoding the serotonin 2A receptor is associated with outcome of antidepressant treatment. *Am. J. Hum. Genet.*, **78**, 804–14.

Melfi, C. A., Croghan, T. W., Hanna, M. P. *et al.* (2000). Racial variation in antidepressant treatment in a Medicaid population. *J. Clin. Psychiatry*, **61**, 16–21.

Morgenstern, H. & Glazer, W. M (1993). Identifying risk factors for tardive dyskinesia among long-term outpatients maintained with neuroleptic medications: results of the Yale Tardive Dyskinesia Study. *Arch. Gen. Psychiatry*, **50**, 723–33.

Okpaku, S., Frazer, A. & Mendels, J. (2005). A pilot study of racial differences in erythrocyte lithium transport. *Am. J. Psychiatry*, **137**, 120–1.

Pi, E. H. & Simpson G. M. (2005). Cross-cultural psychopharmacology: a current clinical perspective. *Psychiatry Serv.*, **56**, 31–3.

Sankar, P. & Kahn, J. (2005). BiDil: Race medicine or race marketing? *Health Affairs*, web exclusive (http://content.healthaffairs.org/cgi/content/abstract/hlthaff.w5.455).

Schillevoort, I., de Boer, A., van der Weide J. *et al.* (2002). Antipsychotic-induced extrapyramidal syndromes and cytochrome P450 2D6 genotype: a case-control study. *Pharmacogenetics*, **12**, 235–40.

Segal, S. P., Bola, J. R. & Watson, M. A. (1996). Race, quality of care, and antipsychotic prescribing practices in psychiatric emergency services. *Psychiatric Serv.*, **47**, 282–6.

Shavers, V. L., Lynch, C. F. & Burmeister, L. F. (2000). Knowledge of the Tuskegee study and its impact on the willingness to participate in medical research studies. *J. Natl. Med. Assoc.*, **92**, 563–72.

Shavers, V. L., Lynch, C. F. & Burmeister, L. F. (2002). Racial differences in factors that influence the willingness to participate in medical research studies. *Ann. Epidemiol.*, **12**, 248–56.

Strickland, T. L., Lin, K. M., Fu, P., Anderson, D. *et al.* (1995). Comparison of lithium ratio between African-American and Caucasian bipolar patients. *Biol. Psychiatry*, **37**, 325–30.

Stroup, T. S., Lieberman, J. A., McEvoy, J. P. *et al.* (2006). Effectiveness of olanzapine, quetiapine, risperidone, and ziprasidone in patients with chronic schizophrenia following discontinuation of a previous atypical antipsychotic. *Am. J. Psychiatry*, **163**, 611–22.

Taylor, A. L., Ziesche, S., Yancy, C. *et al.* (2004). Combination of isosorbide dinitrate and hydralazine in Blacks with heart failure. *N. Engl. J. Med.*, **351**, 2049–57.

Tollefson, G. D., Beasley, C. M., Tran, V. P. *et al.* (1997). Olanzapine versus haloperidol in the treatment of schizophrenia and schizoaffective and schizophreniform disorders: results of an international collaborative trial. *Am. J. Psychiatry*, **154**, 457–65.

Tran, P. T., Lawson, W. B., Andersen, S. *et al.* (1999). Treatment of the African American patient with novel antipsychotic agents. In J. M. Herrara, W. B. Lawson and J. J. Sramek, eds., *Cross-Cultural Psychiatry*. Sussex: John Wiley & Sons.

Trivedi, M. H., Rush A. J., Wisniewski, S. R. *et al.* (2006). STAR *D Study Team. Evaluation of outcomes with citalopram for depression using measurement-based care in STAR *D: implications for clinical practice. *Am. J. Psychiatry*, **163**, 28–40.

US Census (2006). Available at: http://www.census.gov/ [Accessed March 6, 2006].

US Department of Health and Human Services (2001). Mental health: culture, race, and ethnicity – a supplement to mental health: a report of the Surgeon General. Rockville, MD: US Department of Health and Human Services, Substance Abuse and Mental Health Services Administration.

US Food and Drug Administration (2005). FDA approves BiDil heart failure drug for Black patients. Press Release, June 23, 2005. www.fda.gov/bbs/topics/NEWS/2005/NEW01190.html [Accessed October 4, 2005].

Valenstein, M., McCarthy, J. F., Austin, K. L. *et al.* (2006). What happened to lithium? Antidepressant augmentation in clinical settings. *Am. J. Psychiatry*, **163**, 1219–25.

Wendler, D., Kington, R., Madans, J. *et al.* (2006). Are racial and ethnic minorities less willing to participate in health research? *PLoS Med.*, **3**, e19.

# 9

# Complementary medicines in mental disorders

Xin Yu

Modern medicine, called "western medicine" by many non-Western cultures, has taken the leading position in all societies while indigenous medicines either disappear completely or recede to "complementary" status. Indigenous medicine, which was mainstream in the past, is still a principal approach in the management of mental disorders in many cultures. Modern medicine was developed through the exploration of pathology, the deep understanding of dysfunction in certain parts of the body formulated with the knowledge of pathophysiology, pharmacology, molecular biology, genetics, and other medical sciences. On the contrary, almost all complementary medicines rely on the construct of human diseases built on the basis of experience and guided by philosophy. Experience-based medicine applies to a "trial and error" model. The accumulation of successful individual cases leads to the birth of new medication or new therapy. For example, arteannuin was extracted from a plant "Sweet Wormwood Herb" (*Artemisiae annuae*), which was widely grown in northern-western China. Local people used this plant for the treatment of malaria for hundreds of years and this regimen was recorded in a few of Chinese medical books.

Chinese philosophy believes that each object in this universe is composed of two elements: yin and yang. When yang is stronger, the object reflects characteristics such as warm, bright, positive, and so on, when yin is stronger, it manifests cold, dark, negative properties. However, yin and yang are not consistent nor mutually exclusive. The predominance of yin or yang changes over time due to various environmental or internal factors. Yin and yang theory combines with internal components, such as vitality (qi), blood (xue), spirit (shen), and external components, such as cold (han), heat (re), wind (feng), to make up the dialectical diagnostic system of traditional Chinese medicine (TCM).

*Ethno-psychopharmacology: Advances in Current Practice*, eds. C. H. Ng, K.-M. Lin, B. S. Singh and E. Y. K. Chiu. Published by Cambridge University Press. © C. H. Ng, K.-M. Lin, B. S. Singh and E. Y. K. Chiu 2008.

Since mental disorders are variously interpreted as the "stasis of vitality," "ascendance of heat," "confusion of phlegm," "shortage of blood" and so on, therefore the therapeutic strategies are targeting to regulate vitality, clear up heat and phlegm, and to supply blood. However, the achievement in TCM does not parallel the advances in modern psychiatry. First, there is no consistent diagnostic criterion for mental disorders. For example, major depression, which is generally accepted and diagnosed by psychiatrists trained in Western medicine, might be interpreted by as many as 50 dialectical diagnostic categories in TCM. It makes the mutual communication problematic between TCM and Western clinicians, and even among TCM physicians themselves. Second, remedies prescribed by TCM physicians are individually tailored, thus clinical trials on TCM medications, which can meet all good clinical practice requirements, will be difficult to arrange. This is why few traditional medications are able to be approved by drug administration agencies such as the FDA of the US or the SFDA of China (Wang *et al.*, 2004).

Just as TCM, all of the other complementary medicines work mainly in those areas where modern medicine can not produce remarkable or immediate efficacy, such as immunological disease, degenerative diseases, cancer, and mental disorders. Few people will seek alternative resolutions for diseases in which effective treatment is already available, even in the places where complementary medicine is very popular.

Patients tend to believe that "medications from nature" are "non-toxic," "non-addicted," and "non-invasive." Therefore complementary medicines are usually used in common, less severe, and chronic mental disorders such as sleep disorders, neurasthenia, and anxiety disorders. It is also applied in "incurable" conditions, for example dementias, autism, and schizophrenia, when doctors and families have tried desperately all means and finally turned to complementary medicine as the last hope.

Until now, one of the most notable studies on TCM is the effectiveness of electric acupuncture (EA) in the treatment of depressive disorders. Initially, comparative study of EA versus amitriptyline showed equal efficacy for depression while the side-effect profile was more favorable for acupuncture. However, those comparative studies are not able to exclude the placebo effect, since subjects who received acupuncture therapy knew that they were being administered this particular treatment. Luo *et al.* (2003) designed a clinical trial to prove the equal efficacy of EA and fluoxetine in the treatment of major depression, in which placebo effect was diminished by the introduction of sham acupuncture. Subjects were randomly assigned to three groups: EA plus placebo; fluoxetine plus sham EA; placebo plus sham EA. After six weeks, both the EA and fluoxetine therapy groups showed better improvements in terms of reduction of total scores of Hamilton Rating Scale for Depression than that in the placebo group. Side effects assessed by the Asberg Adverse Events rating scale did not show any differences among the three groups.

It is hard for complementary medications to transit into modern medications. First of all, it takes time to extract and identify the active component in natural products. Taking TCM as an example, most of the herb preparations are composed of more than ten different botanic species. Traditional Chinese Medicine physicians believe that the miracle of efficacy comes from the amazing composition of those plants. However, pharmacologists will have the most difficulty in finding the specific pharmacologically active substance in the mixture. Second, complementary medicine usually emphasizes "individualization" when making therapeutic strategy, and there is no option of a fixed-dose, standardized preparation working for everyone. Meanwhile, complementary medicine uses all means to impress patients, including naming the medication as the conqueror of a certain disease, packaging the medication in a symbolic way, and regulating the rituals of the administration of such drugs (such as asking patients to take the medication exactly at midnight, by the water from the first rain of spring, and so on). These habituations make randomized controlled trials (RCT) of complementary medicine almost impossible.

There are a few RCT studies evaluating the efficacy of extracts of herbs in the treatment of psychosis (Zhang & Liu 2001). l-Stepholidine (SPD) is extracted from Japanese stephania root. It was proven to have $D_1$ agonist and $D_2$ antagonist effect in animal studies. Wu *et al.* (2003) reported that SPD showed better efficacy both in positive symptoms and negative symptoms compared to perphenazine in a double-blind randomized trial in 61 hospitalized patients with schizophrenia, while unwanted effects particularly extra-pyramidal symptoms (EPS) in SPD treated patients were much less than in those treated with perphenazine. Although SPD is pharmacologically promising, it lacks large-scale trials to prove its clinical efficacy.

Another example of application of complementary medicine in clinical practice is the use of Huperzine-A in the treatment of Alzheimer's disease (AD). Huperzine-A is an extract from *Huperzia serrata*. It can inhibit the activity of acetylcholine esterase (AchE). In vitro studies indicate that Huperzine-A is stronger than physostigmine, neostigmine, and galantamine in terms of AchE inhibition (Han *et al.*, 2004). In a multicenter study, 202 patients with mild to moderate AD were randomly assigned to either Huperzine-A or placebo group for 12 weeks. The huperzine-A treatment group showed significant improvement compared to placebo in terms of cognition, daily functioning, and psychological-behavioral symptoms (Zhang *et al.*, 2002).

In the above two cases, active components were extracted, identified, and tested both pharmacologically and clinically. Other herb preparations, no matter how long they have been used, are still entities that are pharmacologically unknown. Herbal extracts also need better quality monitoring processes, since active components in plants may vary in different varieties and different seasons. If chemical synthesis is less costly than extraction from plants, herbal medicine will be transformed into more readily available components.

Although there is a common belief that natural herbs do no harm, emergent cases reported that renal failure was associated with chronic use of certain herbal preparations. Another important issue is the interaction between herbs and Western medication. There is a tendency, from that assumption, to neglect the possible side effects induced by the combination of both medications. Drug–drug interactions are listed in the following examples.

- Interference with absorption: when isoniazid is co-administered with borax, plaster, magnet or metal complex, further absorption is prevented.
- Synergy of therapeutic pharmacological effects: St. John's Wort will induce serotonin syndrome when co-administered with SSRIs.
- Synergy of unwanted pharmacological effect: ginseng and its products will inhibit the central nervous system (CNS) when they are applied with luminal, chloral hydrate, or ephedrine, which can increase the release of dopamine, noradrenaline, and serotonin in the CNS thus inducing a "hypertensive crisis" if monoamine oxidase inhibitors (MAOIs) are given simultaneously.
- Interaction with drug metabolism: liquorices, which are the most commonly used herbs in TCM can increase metabolites (e.g., nortriptyline, desipramine, and norclomipramine) of tricyclic antidepressants (TCAs) and may produce more side effects (such as dry mouth, constipation, palpitation, etc.) (Xu, 2004; Zhu & Huang, 2004).

There are some principles in complementary medicine that have lessons for Western medicine.

- The holistic concept: complementary medicines such as TCM do not take symptoms or signs as isolated phenomenon. It is considered that all disorders are induced by the dysfunction of the whole body.
- Assist rather than fight against the therapeutic approach: TCM believes that a change of internal harmonious state is the crucial element in the onset and development of any illness, even in infectious diseases. Thus the main therapeutic approach taken by TCM is to assist the patient to rebuild his or her inner harmony rather than killing foreign invaders.
- Individualized diagnosis and treatment: TCM believes that each individual is unique. Thus the diagnosis and treatment plan can only be made for this particular person. All relevant factors such as his or her lifestyle, physical attributes, and environmental components are taken into account.

Complementary medicine can co-exist with modern medicine. Before a cure is found for mental disorders, complementary medicine can provide additional hope or relief of psychic pain and discomfort for patients and their families in expectation of possible improvement. In those societies where modern medicine is not fully available, complementary medicine is essential to keep people with mental disorders in the role of "patients" rather than that of "criminals" or "the cursed." Physicians trained in Western medicine usually regard medicine that is different from what they learned in medical schools at best as heterodoxy and at worst as superstition. However, recruiting complementary medicine as an ally rather than seeing it as an enemy of modern Western medicine may add to our currently available, but still limited, pharmacological armamentarium.

In the interest of patients whose wellbeing is the physician's paramount priority, an understanding and recognition of the possible, appropriate, and useful role complementary medicine may play in the relief of their suffering, can contribute to a more holistic and comprehensive outcome.

## REFERENCES

Han, H., Li, D. & Zhang, D. (2004). The advances in the treatment of dementias with Chinese traditional medicine. *Zhejiang Journal of Traditional Chinese Medicine*, **11**, 498–9.

Luo, H., Ureil, H., Shen, Y. *et al.* (2003). Comparative study of electroacupuncture and fluoxetine for treatment of depression. *Chinese Journal of Psychiatry*, **36**(4), 215–19.

Wang, J., Huang, Y. & Chen, S . (2004). Advances in the treatment of depression with Chinese traditional medicine. *Traditional Chinese Medicine Research*, **17**(3), 64–5.

Wu, D., Xiung, X., Wang, L. *et al.* (2003). A double-blind comparison trial of l-stepholidine and perphenazine in treatment of schizophrenia. *Chinese Journal of New Drugs and Clinical Remedies*, **22**(3), 155–60.

Xu, G. (2004). Drug–drug interaction between herb medicine and western medicine. *Chinese Remedies and Clinics*, **4**(3), 236–7.

Zhang, M. & Liu, W . (2001). The advances in the treatment of schizophrenia with Chinese traditional medicine. *Journal of Tianjin College of Traditional Chinese Medicine*, **20**(4), 39–41.

Zhang, Z., Wang, X., Chen, Q. *et al.* (2002). Clinical efficacy and safety of huperzine A in treatment of mild to moderate Alzheimer disease, a placebo-controlled, double-blind, randomized trial. *National Medical Journal of China*, **82**(14), 941–5.

Zhu, W. & Huang, X . (2004). Pharmacokinetic changes in the combination of herb medicine and western medicine. *China Pharmacy*, **15**(6), 377–9.

# 10

# Cultural factors and the use of psychotropic medications

Chee H. Ng and Steven Klimidis

## Culture and attitudes towards medications

The prescription and use of medications fundamentally involves a social transaction that carries both symbolic and social meanings based on the interactions between the patient, doctor, and their social environment (Moerman, 1979). Consequently medication uptake and use is considerably influenced by sociocultural factors, ultimately influencing therapeutic benefit, as first surmised by Murphy (1969). Cross-cultural and cross-ethnic differences in drug response are considerable, and beyond explanations based simply on the biological effects of the medication. Sociocultural factors include beliefs and expectations concerning the illness, the treatment and its mechanisms of action, compliance behavior, the role of the social network in using medicines, propensity to placebo effects, and use of alternative or concurrent herbal and other strategies from traditional medicines. The patient's willingness to accept medication is related to cross-cultural variability in drug tolerance and metabolism, as well as past experiences and current beliefs and perceptions held about psychiatric drugs.

Sociocultural, illness, and biological factors affect individual attitudes towards psychotropic medications. Health beliefs or explanatory models, particularly causal attributions regarding the illness and the treatment options afforded within such models, exert a profound influence on patients' attitudes and behavior regarding medications (Smith, Lin & Mendoza, 1993). Such effects can be subtle and can occur during the course of treatment even if there has been initial successful negotiation about the nature of the illness and treatment. In psychiatric illness little research has been leveled at the personal meaning that patients bring to treatment practices such as electro-convulsive therapy (ECT), oral medications, and depot injections, or to the transition between different administrative routes and types of medications.

*Ethno-psychopharmacology: Advances in Current Practice*, eds. C. H. Ng, K.-M. Lin, B. S. Singh and E. Y. K. Chiu. Published by Cambridge University Press. © C. H. Ng, K.-M. Lin, B. S. Singh and E. Y. K. Chiu 2008.

**Table 10.1** Determinants of attitudes towards psychotropic medications

| | |
|---|---|
| Biological | Psychopathology |
| | Illness-related neurocognitive impairment |
| | Current and past experience with medication therapeutic and side effects |
| Psychological | Insight into illness |
| | Illness explanatory models |
| | Beliefs about treatment models |
| | Subjective responses to medication effects |
| | Lack of medical information |
| | Personal meaning of accepting psychiatric treatments |
| Sociocultural | Stigma of psychiatric illness and treatments |
| | Attitudes of family and their support network |
| | Preference of traditional medicines |
| | Sociocultural values and influences |

At the very least that medication is deemed necessary confirms having a condition that is highly stigmatized in many societies, and perhaps more in non-Western (Ng, 1997), and may lead patients to question their self-identity and capabilities in their personal and social roles (Carder, Vuckovic & Green, 2003). Insight into the nature of psychiatric illness in turn affects patients' attitude to medications (David, 1990) and compliance (Ziguras, Klimidis, Lambert *et al.*, 2001).

In addition, the cognitive and behavioral effects of medication may influence attitudes and compliance. For instance, subjective reflection on the unpleasant physical and cognitive side effects of psychotropics is likely to result in negative attitudes and foster non-compliance (Awad, 1993). Attitudes in the patient's social network can influence both the patient's behavior and compliance (Mantonakis, Markidis, Kontaxakis *et al.*, 1985). In sociocentric/collectivist societies, in particular, families play a significant role in decisions about illness and what to do about it. In Chinese groups for example there is substantial family involvement and responsibility in the treatment of those suffering from mental illness (Lin, Miller, Poland *et al.*, 1991). Hence, attitudes to medication and medical treatment in general are complex and involve various dimensions including subjective responses to medications, illness insight, health and treatment beliefs that are embedded within cultural worldviews of the patient and family, and social influences that are subject to cultural determination (see Table 10.1).

The occurrence of placebo response remains largely underestimated and unexplored in Western medicine perhaps due to the narrow focus on biomedical technology (Kleinman, 1988). The impact of symbolic healing is often neglected in clinical trials other than being regarded as a confounding factor or relegated to "non-specific," unmeasured, and poorly understood effects. Nevertheless, in general, the placebo response occurs in at least a third of subjects in the majority of clinical drug trials (Swartzman & Burkell, 1998), suggesting a need to shift the emphasis to understanding how and why "non-specific" factors may contribute to therapeutic benefits. Clinically this implies greater attention to factors, which are summarized below, that affect attitudes and behaviors of individual patients towards medications. It is noteworthy that multicenter clinical drug trials involving numerous ethnic groups and cross-national comparisons suggest that there may be a higher placebo response rate in non-Caucasians (Escobar & Tuason, 1980). The expectations of drug effects are often shaped by the patient's cultural origin and past experiences, and may well play an important role in producing the clinical effects of pharmacotherapy, mediated through symbolic and social mechanisms. Characteristics such as the tablet color and size but also, most importantly, the means of preparation of the medicine appear to influence placebo responses (Buckalew & Coffield, 1982).

The majority of Chinese are still influenced by traditional Chinese medicine concepts and practices. In Chinese societies patients are often expected to take herbal preparations home and to be engaged in their preparation (e.g., mixing and boiling the herbs) before ingestion or application. Such rituals are culturally normative and culturally sanctioned, fit within the cultural worldview of the illness and its treatment, and promote a sense of control over the nature of the medicine (not just its use). These factors may be important in determining and preserving positive attitudes and compliance behavior (Ajzen, 2001; Leventhal, Diefenbach, & Leventhal, 1992) in this culture, but many of these are not prominent aspects in Western medication practices. Many non-Western patients use the "herbal medicine approach," which expects rapid relief, few or no side effects, "static" dose regime, and a simple switch to another medicine if lacking rapid relief. This is incongruent with Western psychopharmacotherapy, which is characterized by gradual improvement, notable side effects, individualized dosages, regular clinical supervision and monitoring, the need for patient education, and combination with psychosocial therapies over variable durations (Westermeyer, 1989).

Concerns about psychotropic side effects, which can vary cross-culturally, often lead to premature cessation of psychotropics. This may be related to different propensities for and values placed on somatic experiences in different cultures. Transcultural research indicates that patients from non-Western cultures are more likely to present with predominantly somatic symptoms of psychiatric disorders (Ng, 1997; Parker, Gladstone & Chee, 2001), as cultural explanatory models and social demands may serve to bias information processing in the various domains of subjective experience (Angel & Thoits, 1987). Several studies have shown that the perception and reporting of side effects are influenced by cultural beliefs

(Lin & Shen, 1991). In a study of lithium side effects, although the side-effect profile was similar to Caucasian patients, Chinese patients showed more concern about fatigue and drowsiness but less concern about polydipsia and polyuria, the latter being regarded as a way of removing toxins from the body, consistent with popular Chinese beliefs (Lee, 1993). Clearly, whether one regards a side effect as deleterious or not (and perhaps worthy or not of reporting to the clinician) is influenced by the meaning attached to the experience.

There are cultural differences in expectations and the interpretations of drug effects, which can significantly influence the acceptance of treatment. East Asian patients commonly perceive that Western medicines are more potent and have greater adverse effects than herbal or traditional therapies (Lee, 1980; Smith, Lin & Mendoza, 1993). Subjective experiences of medication (as opposed to direct pharmacological effects) are clinically important and should not be dismissed or regarded as non-specific. Negative subjective response to neuroleptics are associated with non-compliance and poorer therapeutic outcome (Awad, Hogan, Voruganti *et al.*, 1995; Van Putten & May, 1978), and similarly noted in antidepressant treatment (Priebe, 1987). In cultural contexts where there is already negative attitude towards Western medicines, adverse effects are likely to confirm established beliefs, augment negative attitudes, and promote default in their use.

## Medication compliance in pharmacotherapy

Based essentially on Western literature, which focuses on the individual patient as the principal conduit for treatment, the patient's knowledge about the nature and actions of medications and the attitude towards and interpretation of its effects are central to medication compliance. Despite being widely studied, the issue of non-compliance remains a major problem in clinical practice associated with very high health costs and adverse outcomes. Non-compliance rates in those with psychiatric disorders vary between 25% to 80%, with a high percentage of patients who do not even fill their prescriptions (Fenton, Blyler & Heinssen, 1997). As a general rule, only about a third of patients is compliant with their treatment, another third is partially compliant, and the remainder totally non-compliant. Partial compliance implies not taking prescribed medications at the right dose or taking them at the wrong time, or irregularly, or for the wrong reasons (Wertheimer & Santella, 2003). Sometimes patients may take too much medication in the hope for additional benefits, erroneously assuming that more is better.

Although non-compliance has not been consistently linked with any specific demographic it has been associated with numerous factors related to the illness, patient, clinician, and the medication itself as shown in Table 10.2.

**Table 10.2** Factors related to treatment non-adherence

| Aspects | Factors |
| --- | --- |
| Illness | Symptom severity |
| | Chronicity of illness |
| | Co-morbid medical or psychiatric illness |
| | Impaired cognitive function |
| Patient | Lack of insight |
| | Lack of communication skills |
| | Negative attitudes or false beliefs about medications |
| | Lack of access to appropriate information |
| | Lack of medical knowledge and psychoeducation |
| | Illness explanatory models incongruent to clinician |
| | Patient preference for non-medication treatment (psychotherapy) |
| | Lack of affordability |
| | Barriers to clinical care (e.g., transport) |
| | Cultural and language barriers to care |
| | Lack of social supports (family, friends, or professionals) |
| Clinician | Poor doctor–patient relationship |
| | Complex medication regimen |
| | Lack of expertise or experience with psychotropic drugs |
| | Inadequate time to explore psychosocial needs |
| | Lack of compliance education provided |
| | Inadequate discussion about potential side effects, and duration of treatment |
| | Lacking in flexibility to change regimen in response to side effects |
| | Lack of contingency planning in case of non-compliance |
| Medication | Intolerable side effects |
| | Too expensive |
| | Dosing schedules too complex |
| | Laboratory monitoring required |
| | Lack of efficacy or delay in achieving efficacy |

Adapted from Bourgeois, 2005.

Non-compliance issues appear more prevalent in some non-Western cultures. One study in South Africa revealed non-compliance rates to oral neuroleptics in two-thirds of Black patients and one-half of "colored" patients compared to only one-quarter of Caucasians (Gillis, Trollip, Jakoet *et al.*, 1987). Cultural and communication factors were considered to be significant barriers apart from those related to cost and social factors. Kinzie *et al.* (1987) reported that despite prescribing adequate doses of tricyclic antidepressants (TCAs) to depressed Asian refugees,

61% did not have any TCA in their blood and 24% had very low serum levels. Improvement in compliance rate resulted from better education about the role of medications. Factors associated with non-compliance in migrant patients from non-Western cultures include limited education, lack of understanding of disorders or rationale for treatment, low acculturation or cultural isolation, mistrust of the Western healthcare system, competitive use of traditional remedies, uncertainty in dealing with side effects, and a tendency to cease medication prematurely (Westermeyer, 1989). Premature cessation may be a response to perceptions of early symptom remission or, more commonly, expectations that the medication effects should be more immediate and that the medication is "not working," in addition to the awareness of side effects. Further, the concurrence of physical symptoms in mental disorders such as depression is associated with lower likelihood in starting or completing treatment (Nutting, Post, Smith *et al.*, 2000). This has relevance in Asian and other non-Western patients with high prevalence of somatization, which may take precedence over mood or cognitive symptoms and could lead to greater treatment dropout.

Furthermore, different communication styles in Asian patients, characterized by a less direct and assertive manner, may explain why many patients may readily agree with the treatment plan (in order to please the clinician) yet they do not comply with it (Tung, 1985). On the other hand, due to cultural patterns in social relationships, Asian patients may expect a more authoritarian doctor–patient relationship, often resulting in passive acceptance of treatment but poor understanding of the medication (Lee, 1993). There is poor compliance when there are failures to convey treatment information in a culturally acceptable model, to involve the family unit, and to allocate sufficient time to clarify their expectations and for decision-making. Discords in communication and in conceptualization of illness and therapy are also subject to cultural variation, as are stress levels, nature of social support, and personality styles (Lin, Poland & Silver, 1993). In a study of immigrants with psychosis, greater compliance was evident for patients receiving case management by compatriot bilingual/bicultural clinicians than others, over and above a general cooperative attitude in the patient with the treatment and the negative influence of poor illness insight (Ziguras, Klimidis, Lambert *et al.*, 2001), pointing to the important influences of cultural and linguistic compatibility between the patient and clinician.

Additional strategies for promoting compliance include simplifying dosing, cueing dosing to daily routine, use of a pill dosette box, self-monitoring of symptoms, providing better access to appropriate information, and encouragement of family supervision or involvement. It is also important to address the negative attitudes towards medications, confront any counter-productive beliefs or stigma, and negotiate a culturally acceptable illness concept that is compatible with taking medications. A "good" patient–clinician relationship is important (Day, Bentall, Roberts *et al.*, 2005) but this area requires more research in both Western and especially in non-Western groups where this may be defined quite differently. Within Western groups a physician–patient "partnership" is highlighted as a productive model in dealing with chronic disease, with the underlying assumptions that the role of the doctor is to provide technical assistance to the patient who is expected to take to a self-management role and have strong participation in treatment decision-making. This may be incongruous with cultural expectations of the doctor as an authority (over and beyond his technical knowledge) in many cultural groups. It is also inconsistent with the realities of psychiatric treatment where the problem of involuntary treatment is commonplace and needs to be negotiated carefully (Seale, Chaplin, Lelliott *et al.*, 2006).

## Measurement of attitudes towards psychotropic drugs

Valid and accurate monitoring of attitudes to drug therapy has the potential to influence outcome through the management of negative subjective response and targeted clinical interventions. Several rating instruments have been developed to measure aspects of general attitudes, expectations, and subjective response to medications. One of the most widely used self-report scale in clinical and research settings is the Drug Attitude Inventory (DAI) (Hogan, Awad & Eastwood, 1983). The items are grouped into seven categories including subjective positive, subjective negative, health/illness, physician, control, prevention, and harm. A shorter version (DAI-10) was subsequently developed with ten questions mostly derived from the subjective and negative categories (Awad, Hogan, Voruganti *et al.*, 1995). Other instruments to measure various dimensions of attitudes and compliance have been developed and validated against the DAI. For instance, the Attitudes towards Neuroleptic Treatment was designed to measure attitudes, expectation, and insight in relation to drugs both before and after treatment (Kampman, Lehtinen, Lassila *et al.*, 2000). Another scale is the Medication Adherence Rating Scale, which was developed by combining the DAI and the Medication Adherence Questionnaire (Morisky, Green & Levine, 1986). This scale was designed to improve the detection and measurement of drug compliance (Thompson, Kulkarni & Sergejew, 2000). More recently, another scale known as the Personal Evaluation of Transitions in Treatment has been validated to measure subjective aspects (personal response, adherence, and quality of life) perceived during the course of drug treatment in schizophrenia (Voruganti & Awad, 2002). It is noteworthy that none of these approaches to measurement has been designed for application specific to non-Western groups.

The Medication Attitude Scale (MAS) was developed by the authors as a self-rating scale to quantify both general and culturally based attitudes towards psychotropic medications. Building from the established DAI that measures generic attitudes to neuroleptic treatment, this new scale has incorporated the assessment of attitudes and perception of drug effects among patients from different cultures. The psychometric properties of the scale were determined by field testing in patients with different psychiatric disorders and ethnic backgrounds. The 25 items consist of brief simple statements that are scored on a four-point scale measuring relevance to the patient, labeled "completely true," "mostly true," "mostly false," and "completely false." This allows assessment of the degree that the views and attitudes are held about the medications rather than just a true/false dichotomy, and is simple to use in patients with both acute and chronic psychiatric problems.

From the data of a preliminary study, the MAS is reliable, valid, and sensitive to change across different diagnostic groups and cultural backgrounds. The inclusion of culturally appropriate items with an expanded scoring scale may increase the level of utility and sensitivity that can be used in a wide range of clinical settings. Importantly, the MAS comprises two factors that are relatively independent, measuring positive and negative attitudes towards medications, enabling examination of the relative contribution of these to medication acceptance and compliance. Indeed patients can be regarded to have a combination of positive and negative attitudes towards medications as there appears to be a subjective weighting of perceived harms against perceived benefits guiding their acceptance of the medication (Horne, Graupner, Frost *et al.*, 2004; Horne & Weinman, 1999). This two-factor model of attitudes is consistent with a wider body of work examining attitudinal ambivalence, which is linked to inconsistency in behavioral outcomes (Ajzen, 2001).

In our study (Ng & Klimidis, submitted), 51 Asian patients and 36 Caucasian patients, who in one group met DSM-IV criteria for chronic schizophrenia and in another group, criteria for major depressive disorder, were treated with clozapine and sertraline respectively (Ng, Norman, Naing *et al.*, 2006; Ng, Chong, Lambert *et al.*, 2005). There was a significant race effect on the negative scale ($p = 0.007$) and total scale ($p = 0.003$) but not the positive scale ($p = 0.09$) as shown in Figure 10.1. The mean negative subscale scores indicate that the Asian subjects (X = 2.30) had more negative attitudes to medications than Caucasian patients (X = 1.97), consistent with cross-cultural literature. No significant difference in total MAS scores was observed in relation to the variables of age, gender, or diagnosis. Although there was lack of correlation between the total scores of the MAS and a side-effects scale ($r = -0.13$, $p = 0.22$), side-effect scores weakly correlated with the negative scale ($r = 0.24$, $p = 0.03$). Asian patients had less positive attitudes towards medications compared with Caucasian patients, despite having fewer side effects. This may reflect cultural differences on the value placed on medications and the expectation of their effects, although other factors such as illness course, experience

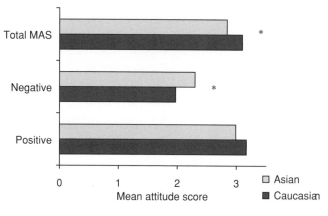

MAS = Medication attitude scale; *ANOVA p < 0.01

Figure 10.1  Effect of ethnicity on Medication Attitude Scale total and subscale scores

of previous side effects, and need for blood monitoring may also influence attitudes. Treatment itself may exert a significant attitudinal change as indicated in the sertraline sample we examined. Here, depression ratings were significantly lower by the end of the six-week treatment trial and there were concurrent increases in positive attitudes and decreases in negative attitudes. Further, less clinical improvement was related negatively with positive attitudes as measured by the MAS at the end of the trial.

## Summary

Sociocultural factors significantly contribute to differences in drug response. Different cultures experience disease states in different ways and effectively may have different expression of illness with the same disease. Cultural and other traditional medicines translate into popular local conceptions of disease, foster different explanatory models for them, and determine the nature of illness that is relevant to treat. Peoples of different cultures experience their own medicines in habitual ways that may not align well to the Western allopathic tradition. Western medicines may be subject to different beliefs by different cultural groups affecting their attitudes towards them, and where these are substantially discrepant practices from their traditional practices this may foster a lack of their acceptance and failure in compliance. It is important, in addition to other considerations, that clinical practice extends to understanding the symbolic and transactional nature of the process of prescribing and using medications, especially when negotiating treatment in patients from non-Western cultures. Identifying negative attitudes, perception, and the meanings of medications and medication practices within the clinical context may help to improve therapeutic alliance, compliance, and treatment completion. Assessment of attitudes towards medications that are influenced by cultural beliefs and views are hence informative for planning appropriate interventions and for optimizing treatment outcomes in patients from different cultures.

# REFERENCES

Ajzen, I. (2001). Nature and operation of attitudes. *Annu. Rev. Psychol.*, **52**, 27–58.

Angel, R. & Thoits, P. (1987). The impact of culture on the cognitive structure of illness. *Cult. Med. Psychiatry*, **11**, 465–94.

Awad, A. G. (1993). Subjective response to neuroleptics in schizophrenia. *Schizophr. Bull.*, **19**, 609–18.

Awad, A. G., Hogan, T. P., Voruganti, L. N. & Heslegrave, R. J. (1995). Patient's subjective experiences on antipsychotic medications: implications for outcome and quality of life. *Int. Clin. Psychopharmacol.*, **10**, 123–32.

Bourgeois, J. A. (2005). Compliance with psychiatric treatment in primary care: review and strategies. *Prim. Psychiatry*, **12**, 40–7.

Buckalew, L. W. & Coffield, K. E. (1982). Drug expectations associated with perceptual characteristics. *Percept. Mot. Skills*, **55**, 915–18.

Carder, P. C., Vuckovic, N. & Green, C. A. (2003). Negotiating medications: patient perceptions of long-term medication use. *J. Clin. Pharm. Ther.*, **28**, 409–17.

David, A. S. (1990). Insight and psychosis. *Br. J. Psychiatry*, **156**, 798–808.

Day, J. C., Bentall, R. P., Roberts, C. *et al.* (2005). Attitudes toward antipsychotic medication. *Arch. Gen. Psychiatry*, **62**, 717–24.

Escobar, J. I. & Tuason, V. B. (1980). Antidepressant agents: a cross-cultural study. *Psychopharmacol. Bull.*, **16**, 49–52.

Fenton, W. S., Blyler, C. R. & Heinssen, R. K. (1997). Determinants of medication compliance in schizophrenia: empirical and clinical findings. *Schizophr. Bull.*, **23**, 637–51.

Gillis, L. S., Trollip, D., Jakoet, A. & Holden, T. (1987). Non-compliance with psychotropic medication. *S. Afr. Med. J.*, **72**(9), 602–6.

Hogan, T. P., Awad, A. G. & Eastwood, R. (1983). A self-report scale predictive of drug compliance in schizophrenics: reliability and discriminative validity. *Psychol. Med.*, **13**, 177–83.

Horne, R. & Weinman, J. (1999). Patients' beliefs about prescribed medicines and their role in adherence to treatment in chronic physical disease. *J. Psychosom. Res.*, **47**(6), 555–67.

Horne, R., Graupner, L., Frost, S. *et al.* (2004). Medicine in a multi-cultural society: the effect of cultural background on beliefs about medications. *Soc. Sci. Med.*, **59**, 1307–13.

Kampman, O., Lehtinen, K., Lassila, V. *et al.* (2000). Attitudes towards neuroleptic treatment: reliability and validity of the Attitudes towards Neuroleptic Treatment (ANT) questionnaire. *Schizophr. Res.*, **45**, 223–34.

Kinzie, J. D., Leung, P., Boehnlein, J. K. & Fleck, J. (1987). Antidepressant blood levels in Southeast Asians. Clinical and cultural implications. *J. Nerv. Ment. Dis.*, **175**(8), 480–5.

Kleinman, A. (1988). *Rethinking Psychiatry*. New York: Free Press.

Lee, R. P. L. (1980). Perceptions and uses of Chinese medicine among the Chinese in Hong Kong. *Cult. Med. Psychiatry*, **4**, 345–75.

Lee, S. (1993). Side effect of chronic lithium therapy in Hong Kong Chinese: an ethnopsychiatric perspective. *Cult. Med. Psychiatry*, **17**, 301–20.

Leventhal, H., Diefenbach, M. & Leventhal, E. A. (1992). Illness cognition: using common sense to understand treatment adherence and affect cognition interactions. *Cogn. Ther. Res.*, **16**, 143–63.

Lin, K.-M. & Shen, W. W. (1991). Pharmacotherapy for Southeast Asian psychiatric patients. *J. Nerv. Ment. Dis.*, **179**, 346–50.

Lin, K.-M., Miller, M. H., Poland, R. E., Nuccio, I. & Yamaguchi, M. (1991). Ethnicity and family involvement in the treatment of schizophrenic patients. *J. Nerv. Ment. Dis.*, **179**, 631–3.

Lin, K.-M., Poland, R. E. & Silver, B. (1993). Overview: the interface between psychobiology and ethnicity. In K. M. Lin, R. E. Poland and G. Nakasaki, eds., *Psychopharmacology and Psychobiology of Ethnicity*. Washington, DC: American Psychiatric Press, pp. 11–35.

Mantonakis, J., Markidis, M., Kontaxakis, V. & Liakos, A. (1985). A scale for detection of negative attitudes towards medication among relatives of schizophrenic patients. *Acta Psychiatr. Scand.*, **71**, 186–9.

Moerman, D. E. (1979). Anthropology of symbolic healing. *Curr. Anthropology*, **20**, 59–80.

Morisky, D. E., Green, L. W. & Levine, D. M. (1986). Concurrent and predictive validity of a self-reported measure of medication adherence. *Med. Care*, **24**, 67–74.

Murphy, H. B. M. (1969). Ethnic variations in drug response. *Transcultural Psychiatric Research Review*, **6**, 6–23.

Ng, C. (1997). The stigma of mental illness in Asian cultures. *Aust. N. Z. J. Psychiatry*, **31**, 382–90.

Ng, C., Chong, S. A., Lambert, T. *et al.* (2005). An interethnic comparison study of clozapine dosage, clinical response and plasma levels. *Int. Clin. Psychopharmacol.*, **20**, 163–8.

Ng, C., Norman, T., Naing, K. O. *et al.* (2006). A comparison study of sertraline dosages and response in Chinese versus Caucasian patients. *J. Int. Clin. Psychopharmacol.*, **21**, 87–92.

Nutting, P. A., Post, K., Smith, J., Werner, J. J. & Elliot, C. (2000). Competing demands from physical problems: effect on initiating and completing depression care over 6 months. *Arch. Fam. Med.*, **9**, 1959–64.

Parker, G., Gladstone, G. & Chee, K.-T. (2001). Depression in the planet's largest ethnic group: the Chinese. *Am. J. Psychiatry*, **158**, 857–64.

Priebe, S. (1987). Early subjective reactions predicting outcome of hospital treatment in depressive patients. *Acta Psychiatr. Scand.*, **76**, 134–8.

Seale, C., Chaplin, R., Lelliott, P. & Quirk, A. (2006). Sharing decisions in consultations involving anti-psychotic medication: a qualitative study of psychiatrists' experiences. *Soc. Sci. Med.*, **62**, 2861–73.

Smith, M., Lin, K. M. & Mendoza, R. (1993). Non-biological issues affecting psycho-pharmacotherapy: cultural considerations. In K. M. Lin, R. E. Poland and G. Nakasaki, eds., *Psychopharmacology and Psychobiology of Ethnicity*. Washington DC: American Psychiatric Press, pp. 37–58.

Swartzman, L. C. & Burkell, J. (1998). Expectations and the placebo effect in clinical drug trials: why we should not turn a blind eye to unblinding, and other cautionary notes. *Clin. Pharmacol. Ther.*, **64**, 1–7.

Thompson, K., Kulkarni, J. & Sergejew, A. (2000). Reliability and validity of a new Medication Adherence Rating Scale (MARS) for the psychoses. *Schizophr. Res.*, **42**, 241–7.

Tung, T. M. (1985). Psychiatric care for Southeast Asian patients: how different is different? In T. Owan, B. Bliatout, K. M. Lin *et al.*, eds., *Southeast Asian Mental Health: Treatment, Prevention, Services and Research*. Rockville, MD: National Institute of Mental Health.

Van Putten, T. & May, P. R. A. (1978). Subjective response as a predictor of outcome in pharmacotherapy. *Arch. Gen. Psychiatry*, **35**, 477–80.

Voruganti, L. N. P. & Awad, A. G. (2002). Personal evaluation of transitions in treatment (PETiT): a scale to measure subjective aspects of antipsychotic drug therapy in schizophrenia. *Schizophr. Res.*, **56**, 37–46.

Wertheimer, A. I. & Santella, T. M. (2003). Medication compliance research: still far to go. *J. of Applied Res. in Clin. and Exp. Therapeutics*, **3**(3), (http://jrnlappliedresearch.com/articles/Vol3Iss3/Wertheimer.htm).

Westermeyer, J. (1989). Somatotherapies. In J. H. Gold, ed., *Psychiatric Care of Migrants: A Clinical Guide*. Washington: American Psychiatric Press, pp. 139–68.

Ziguras, S. J., Klimidis, S., Lambert, T. J. R. & Jackson, A. C. (2001). Determinants of anti-psychotic medication compliance in a multicultural population. *Community Ment. Health J.*, **37**(3), 273–83.

# 11

# Outpatient prescribing practices in Asian countries

Pichet Udomratn and Chee H. Ng

## Introduction

Every country has its differences in the characteristics of psychiatric practice including those relating to prescribing psychotropic drugs. In Asian countries only limited data is available. Most of the earlier data involved Asian refugees or Asian patients born in Western countries and the results were also inconsistent (Bond, 1991). However, Asia covers a large geographical area and diverse populations with different physical features, cultural backgrounds, and dietary habits. The socioeconomic differences in Asian countries also have implications on the number of psychiatrists and mental health workers, and infrastructure for mental health services. A review of outpatients prescribing patterns hence can add to our understanding of important systemic and cultural determinants of psychotropic prescription in the management of major mental disorders. Furthermore, prescribing practice in outpatients services are reflective of real-life clinical settings and long-term exposure to psychotropics affecting patients.

## Antipsychotics prescribing

Reports on prescribing psychotropic practice have mostly comprised antipsychotics in the treatment of schizophrenia and major psychoses. Studies can be broadly divided into "self-reported" questionnaires of prescribing habit or "revealed" data of actual prescription via for example an audit of psychotropic drug usage. An example of the former comes from a questionnaire given to practicing Asian psychiatrists after reading a case vignette of a 28-year-old unmarried businessman with a first episode of paranoid schizophrenia (Udomratn, 1999). The average daily dose of haloperidol that would be prescribed following the first week in the absence of any serious side effects was compared between psychiatrists across Asia.

*Ethno-psychopharmacology: Advances in Current Practice*, eds. C. H. Ng, K.-M. Lin, B. S. Singh and E. Y. K. Chiu. Published by Cambridge University Press. © C. H. Ng, K.-M. Lin, B. S. Singh and E. Y. K. Chiu 2008.

**Table 11.1** Dosage of haloperidol (mg/day) prescribed by psychiatrists in Southeast and East Asian countries

| Country | N | Mean ± S.D. mg/d | Percentage of respondents | | | | | |
| --- | --- | --- | --- | --- | --- | --- | --- | --- |
| | | | <6 mg/d | 6–10 mg/d | 11–15 mg/d | 16–20 mg/d | 21–30 mg/d | >30 mg/d |
| Thailand | 98 | $14.1 \pm 6.9$ | 2.0 | 39.8 | 33.7 | 17.4 | 6.1 | 1.0 |
| Malaysia | 23 | $12.8 \pm 5.7$ | 8.7 | 43.5 | 30.4 | 13.0 | 4.4 | 0 |
| Singapore | 13 | $12.2 \pm 4.9$ | 7.7 | 46.1 | 30.8 | 15.4 | 0 | 0 |
| Taiwan | 93 | $9.6 \pm 4.9^a$ | 21.5 | 58.1 | 7.5 | 11.8 | 1.1 | 0 |
| Hong Kong | 52 | $9.9 \pm 4.5^b$ | 25.0 | 51.9 | 13.5 | 9.6 | 0 | 0 |

[a] Thailand cf. Taiwan $p \leq 0.0001$
[b] Thailand cf. Hong Kong $p \leq 0.0001$

**Table 11.2** Time to switching from haloperidol to a second antipsychotic drug

| Country | N | Percentage of respondents who will switch after ($x$ days) | | | | |
| --- | --- | --- | --- | --- | --- | --- |
| | | <8 | 8–14 | 15–21 | 22–35 | >35 |
| Thailand | 98 | 8.1 | 18.4 | 25.5 | 33.7 | 14.3 |
| Malaysia | 23 | 8.7 | 26.0 | 13.1 | 39.1 | 13.1 |
| Singapore | 13 | 30.7 | 23.1 | 23.1 | 23.1 | 0 |
| Taiwan | 93 | 10.7 | 25.8 | 10.7 | 35.6 | 17.2 |
| Hong Kong | 52 | 7.8 | 40.4 | 9.6 | 21.1 | 21.1 |

Psychiatrists in Southeast Asia such as Thailand, Malaysia, and Singapore would prescribe 12–14 mg/day of haloperidol while East Asian psychiatrists would prescribe a smaller dose of 9–10 mg/day. The average dose range of haloperidol of 6–10 mg/day was the most commonly prescribed dosage (see Table 11.1).

In terms of the time to switching from haloperidol to the second antipsychotic in the event of non-response, it was found that psychiatrists in Singapore and Hong Kong tended to shift earlier, switch between one to two weeks, while psychiatrists in Taiwan, Malaysia, and Thailand would wait for three to five weeks (see Table 11.2). The reason for this is unclear but factors in relation to drug affordability, family expectation, and prescribing culture could be relevant. As this study was done during the mid 1990s, the most common choices of the second neuroleptic were trifluoperazine and chlorpromazine among psychiatrists in these countries.

Apart from conducting the survey before the availability of second-generation antipsychotics (SGAs), other limitations of this study included the requirement of haloperidol as the first choice rather than allowing psychiatrists to choose their preferred neuroleptic. Further, the questionnaire did not seek the reason for the choice of the second drug.

A recent study within six East Asian countries/territories showed wide variations in types of antipsychotics prescribed (Chong *et al.*, 2004). However, the study was conducted in inpatient mental health facilities and will be described further in the next chapter. Even on comparing the outpatient data from Prince of Songkla University Hospital in southern Thailand (Udomratn *et al.*, 2004), it was found that Southeast Asian countries like Singapore (3.6%) and Thailand (13.1%) had a lower prescription rate of SGA compared with East Asian countries/territories such as China (51.3%), Taiwan (42.3%), Hong Kong (35.2%), Korea (27.1%), and Japan (21.5%). Moreover, data taken from different hospitals within the same country may also show differences. An example in Korea where the outpatients prescription for patients with schizophrenia in Seoul National University Hospital found that 88.1% of 825 patients received SGAs (Kwon *et al.*, 2003) which is considerably the highest.

The dosage of clozapine appears to be lower in Asian compared to Caucasian patients. Singaporean patients with schizophrenia received a mean daily dose of 169 mg/day compared with 408 mg/day for the Canadian subjects (Chong *et al.*, 2000) whereas Thai patients received mean doses of 174 mg/day. One study investigated clozapine dosage, plasma clozapine and metabolite levels, and clinical and side effects in Singaporean versus Australian patients with chronic schizophrenia who were on stable maintenance treatment. Although Singaporean patients received significantly lower mean clozapine dose (176 mg/day) than the Australian group (433 mg/day, $p < 0.001$), the plasma clozapine levels were similar between both groups (Ng *et al.*, 2005). One likely explanation was that Asian patients seemed to have significantly lower clozapine clearance compared to Caucasian patients.

The cross-national prescribing database using the same methodology provided a useful and valid comparison of patterns of prescribing psychotropic medications in mental health services in Australia, Thailand, and Malaysia (Ng *et al.*, submitted). The study was carried out in three outpatient mental health centres in North Western Mental Health (NWMH) in Melbourne (September to November 2002), Prince of Songkla University Hospital in Hat Yai (January to March 2003), and Hospital Kuala Lumpur (January to March 2003). The proportions of outpatients treated with a primary diagnosis of a psychotic illness were 91%, 41%, and 75% in the Australian, Thai, and Malaysian samples respectively. Considering psychotropic prescriptions in schizophrenia alone, the majority of patients were prescribed antipsychotics: Australia (93.7%), Thailand (92.9%), and Malaysia (97.7%).

**Table 11.3** Comparison of antipsychotic prescribing for patients with schizophrenia

| | Australia | | Thailand | | Malaysia | |
|---|---|---|---|---|---|---|
| | N | % | N | % | N | % |
| FGAs[a] | 57 | 5.7 | 232 | 75.3 | 1256 | 79.2 |
| Chlorpromazine | 33 | 3.3 | 49 | 15.9 | 461 | 29.1 |
| Haloperidol | 3 | 0.3 | 22 | 7.1 | 386 | 24.3 |
| Perphenazine | – | – | 145 | 47.1 | 68 | 4.3 |
| Thioridazine | – | – | 15 | 4.9 | 236 | 14.9 |
| SGAs[a] | 683 | 68.3 | 45 | 14.6 | 249 | 15.7 |
| Clozapine | 230 | 23.0 | 30 | 9.7 | 25 | 1.6 |
| Olanzapine | 285 | 28.5 | 6 | 1.9 | 49 | 3.1 |
| Risperidone | 133 | 13.3 | 9 | 2.9 | 82 | 5.2 |
| Depot antipsychotics[a] | 303 | 30.3 | 46 | 14.9 | 794 | 50.1 |
| Flupenthixol | 118 | 11.8 | 22 | 7.1 | 350 | 22.1 |
| Fluphenazine | 34 | 3.4 | – | – | 436 | 27.5 |
| Zuclopenthixol | 121 | 12.1 | 24 | 7.8 | 7 | 0.4 |
| Antidotes | 146 | 14.6 | 198 | 64.3 | 936 | 59.0 |
| Benzhexol | 10 | 1.0 | 198 | 64.3 | 934 | 58.9 |
| Benztropine | 136 | 13.6 | – | – | – | – |
| Polypharmacy[b] | 136 | 13.6 | 65 | 21.1 | 754 | 47.5 |
| Depot alone | 213 | 22.7 | 17 | 5.9 | 56 | 3.6 |
| Depot and oral | 90 | 9.6 | 29 | 10.1 | 738 | 47.6 |
| Oral alone | 588 | 62.8 | 204 | 71.3 | 740 | 47.7 |
| Oral and oral | 46 | 4.9 | 36 | 12.6 | 16 | 1.0 |
| **Total** | 1000 | 100 | 308 | 100 | 1586 | 100 |

[a] only individual drugs used in >10% of any population are listed
[b] >1 antipsychotic

There were large differences found in the psychiatric outpatient prescribing patterns between these countries. Table 11.3 compares the types and patterns of antipsychotic and antidote medications used for patients with schizophrenia in the three centers. Significantly higher proportions of Thai and Malaysian patients with schizophrenia received first-generation antipsychotics (FGAs) compared with patients in Australia (p < 0.001). In contrast, a significantly higher proportion of Australian patients were on SGA compared with Thai and Malaysian patients (p < 0.001). The center in Malaysia had the highest rate of depot use compared with Thailand and NWMH (p < 0.001). The most common antipsychotics prescribed are shown in Table 11.3.

**Table 11.4** Comparison of antipsychotic dosages in CPZe (mean ± SD, range) for patients with schizophrenia only

|  | Australia | Thailand | Malaysia |
| --- | --- | --- | --- |
| Overall (mg/day) | 439.8 ± 265.2 (10–1700) | 254.7 ± 190.7 (10–1650) | 422.8± 311.9 (15–1800) |
| FGAs (mg/day) | 173.2 ± 145.6 (10–750) | 249.6 ± 191.7 (10–1500) | 359.5 ± 279.7 (12.5–1500) |
| SGAs (mg/day) | 449.0 ± 248.0 (15–1264) | 182.3 ± 97.6 (25–450) | 278.0 ± 133.8 (50–800) |
| Depots (mg/day) | 318.9 ± 220.4 (30–1680) | 146.1 ± 81.7 (37.5–600) | 169.5 ± 93.6 (25–600) |

A significantly higher proportion of Thai and Malaysian patients were given an antidote compared with NWMH patients ($p < 0.001$). This may possibly be due to the high rate of FGA use associated with greater extra-pyramidal symptoms. The rate of polypharmacy (patients on more than one antipsychotic concurrently) was significantly higher in Malaysia compared with Australia and Thailand ($p < 0.001$). This was primarily attributed to the greater tendency to prescribe a depot and oral combination in Malaysia to patients with schizophrenia. Another reason for polypharmacy seen in Asian countries may be related to cultural concepts of traditional medicine and local belief that a combination of drugs is more effective (Philips *et al.*, 1997). This parallels traditional medicinal approach of using a mixture of herbal ingredients, which is translated to polypharmacy (Binder *et al.*, 1987). Asian psychiatrists also believe that use of multiple antipsychotics could reduce cost and enhance antipsychotic effect (Chong *et al.*, 2000). The varying patterns of antipsychotic use between centers suggest that other systemic and local factors are important in determining prescribing habits.

The overall mean chlorpromazine-equivalents per day (CPZe) dose prescribed differed significantly, with lower dosing in Thailand compared with Malaysia and Australia ($p < 0.001$) (see Table 11.4). Pairwise comparisons revealed that the mean typical antipsychotic dose was significantly higher in Malaysia compared with Thailand ($p < 0.001$) and NWMH ($p < 0.001$). There were significant differences observed ($p < 0.001$) while comparisons of the mean atypical antipsychotic dose showed that Australia was significantly higher compared with Thailand ($p < 0.001$) and Malaysia ($p < 0.001$).

Differences have been found cross-nationally in the treatment of psychotic disorders in terms of types, dosage, and co-prescription of antipsychotics. A major factor that affects the prescription of SGAs in most of the Asian countries is the cost of medication. In most Asian countries, SGAs cost about 10 to 60 times more than FGAs. For example, the price of the original SGA in Thailand (risperidone 2 mg) is eight times higher than the generic clozapine 100 mg and is 74 times higher than the generic haloperidol 5 mg. Hence, the prescribing patterns are strongly influenced by whether SGAs have been approved under the national or hospital pharmaceutical benefits schemes, which will affect out-of-pocket costs for patients and families. Although clinical and biological factors are important determinants in medication prescription, health systems, economics, and culture are equally crucial factors in prescribing patterns.

## Antidepressant prescribing

Compared to antipsychotics, there are even fewer studies on the prescribing patterns of antidepressants done in Asian countries. Pi *et al.* (1985) conducted a survey of psychotropic prescribing practices reported by psychiatrists in 29 medical schools in 9 Asian countries. Daily dose range of tricyclic antidepressants (TCAs) such as amitriptyline, imipramine, and nortriptyline in Asian countries was comparable to the practice in USA. This is despite differences found between Asian and non-Asian populations in the pharmacokinetics of TCAs (Pi *et al.*, 1993). A questionnaire on the practical prescribing approaches in mood disorders administered to 298 Japanese psychiatrists was reported by Oshima *et al.* (1999). As first-line treatment, the majority of respondents chose newer TCAs or non-TCAs for moderate depression and older TCAs for severe depression. Combination of antidepressants and anxiolytics was preferred in moderate depression, while an antidepressant and antipsychotic combination was common in severe psychotic depression. Surprisingly, sulpiride was the most favored drug for dysthymia. In a naturalistic, prospective follow-up of 95 patients with major depression in Japan, the proportion of patients receiving 125 mg/day or less of imipramine was 69% at one month and 67% at six months (Furukawa *et al.*, 2000).

In East London where there are large populations of South Asian residents and general practitioners (GP), the antidepressant prescribing rates were studied. Prescribing rates for antidepressants have almost doubled over five years, the greatest increase being for selective serotonin re-uptake inhibitors (SSRIs). There were significant differences in prescribing practices and rates between UK-trained GPs and South Asian-trained GPs. The highest rates of antidepressant prescribing was reported in UK-trained GPs and in practices with low proportions of South Asian patients. The rate of antidepressant prescribing in South Asian-trained doctors was low regardless of the ethnic composition of the GP practice patients. Reasons for these differences are uncertain, but may be related to differences in the explanatory model for presenting symptoms and management strategies, which rely less on a biomedical paradigm (Hull *et al.*, 2005).

A recent study compared the differences in dosage and steady state plasma concentrations of sertraline, in Chinese versus Caucasian depressed outpatients.

Chinese depressed patients appeared to require lower dosages, with consequently lower plasma concentrations of sertraline compared to Caucasian patients to achieve clinical efficacy (Ng *et al.*, 2006). Again, this finding has supported the fact that Asian patients, especially Chinese, need lower doses of antidepressant drugs than their Western counterparts.

## Anxiolytics and hypnotics prescribing

Benzodiazepines (BZDs) are very frequently prescribed by internists and psychiatrists for the treatment of anxiety symptoms (mainly related to generalized anxiety disorder and psychosomatic disorders) or insomnia. In Asian countries, BZDs are among the most frequently prescribed psychotropic drugs and inappropriate use is also not uncommon. In the survey of psychiatrists in medical schools in Asian countries, the daily dose range of benzodiazepine was higher than in the USA (Pi *et al.*, 1985). In a study from Japan, more than half of the psychiatric outpatients received anxiolytics or hypnotics for basic symptomatic management (Yamawaki, 1999). The type of BZDs most commonly prescribed also varies, for example in Japan thienodiazepine was most often used (Yamawaki, 1999) while in Taiwan the most popular sleep medication for elderly outpatients was lorazepam, followed by zolpidem (Huang & Lai, 2005). In Thailand, a survey among GPs found that the usage of BZDs was high for several conditions including anxiety/insomnia (93%), panic disorder (78%), depression (47%), essential hypertension (27%), and uncomplicated low back pain (18%). About 46% of the GPs acknowledged that they had used BZDs excessively over the past year. Their reasons for over-prescribing included lack of time, lack of knowledge and skills, attention to doctor–patient relationship (i.e., patient demand), lack of alternative treatment to BZDs, and cost saving (Srisurapanont *et al.*, 2005).

Using the insurance computerized data set in Taiwan, the annual consumption of psychotropics was analyzed for the general population in 2003. The one-year prevalence rate of BZD use was 18.63% for the whole sample and 41.8% in those 65 years and older, with 25.53% of the latter taking long-acting BZDs. Females also consumed more BZDs than males in all of the age groups. The defined daily dose per 1000 inhabitants per day was 35.74. The top most frequent prescribers were internists (29.41%), psychiatrists (18.11%), and general practitioners (15.91%). For outpatient prescriptions, 18.87% of the users were written more than one BZD prescription. Those prescribed BZDs also had higher medical service utilization than the general population (26.5 vs.14.2 outpatient clinic visits /person/year). The authors concluded that given the rising prevalence of BZD use, the relevant sociodemographic, clinical, cost, and health outcome factors need to be further explored (Wu *et al.*, 2007).

## Summary

The psychotropic prescribing pattern in outpatient services across different countries varies considerably. Several studies have shown that Asian patients with psychiatric disorders are treated with lower doses of psychotropic drugs than other ethnic groups to achieve a clinical response. Although clinical factors and inter-ethnic differences in drug metabolism may contribute to the differences, prescription habits related to non-clinical factors also play a large role. Factors influencing the prescription of psychotropic drugs include the medical prescribing culture, as well as the availability of medications. Patients' beliefs and attitudes regarding both the cause of illness and the role of the doctor are important in the prescription and acceptance of medication by Asians. Systemic influences on prescribing habits may include the mental health service systems, support structures, prescribing policies, clinical guidelines, drug availability, budgetary restrictions, and drug benefit schemes. Across the Asia-Pacific region, new and modern psychotropic medications are not equally available or prescribed to a large proportion of patients with mental disorders for whom they are indicated. Such pharmaco-economic consequences must be considered when comparing pattern of usage between high-income versus low-income countries. Future studies are needed to explore the sociocultural, economic, and systemic factors.

## REFERENCES

Binder, R. L., Kazamatsuri, H., Hishimura, T. *et al.* (1987). Tardive dyskinesia and antipsychotic-induced parkinsonism in Japan. *Am. J. Psychiatry*, **144**(11), 1494–6.

Bond, W. S. (1991). Ethnicity and psychrotropic drugs. *Clin. Pharm.*, **10**(6), 467–70.

Chong, M. Y., Tan, C. H., Fujii, S. *et al.* (2004). Antipsychotic drug prescription for schizophrenia in East Asia: rationale for change. *Psychiatry Clin. Neurosci.*, **58**(1), 61–7.

Chong, S. A., Remington, G. J., Lee, N. & Mahendran, R. (2000). Contrasting clozapine prescribing patterns in the east and west? *Ann. Acad. Med. Singapore*, **29**(1), 75–8.

Furukawa, T. A., Kitamura, T. & Takahashi, K. (2000). Treatment received by depressed patients in Japan and its determinants: naturalistic observation from multi-center collaborative follow-up study. *J. Affect. Disord.*, **60**(3), 173–9.

Huang, W. F. & Lai, I. C. (2005). Patterns of sleep – related medications prescribed to elderly outpatients with insomnia in Taiwan. *Drugs Aging*, **22**(11), 957–65.

Hull, S. A., Aquino, P. & Cotter, S. (2005). Explaining variation in antidepressant prescribing rates in east London: a cross sectional study. *Fam. Pract.*, **22**(1), 37–42.

Kwon, J. S., Kim, E. T., Ha, T. H. *et al.* (2003). Drug prescribing patterns of outpatients with schizophrenia in a university hospital. *J. Korean Neuropsychiatr. Assoc.*, **42**(6), 683–90.

Ng, C. H., Chong, S. A., Lambert, T. *et al.* (2005). An inter-ethnic comparison study of clozapine dosage, clinical response and plasma levels. *Int. Clin. Psychopharmacol.*, **20**(3), 163–8.

Ng, C. H., Norman, T. R., Naing, K. O. *et al.* (2006). A comparative study of sertraline dosages, plasma concentrations, efficacy and adverse reactions in Chinese versus Caucasian patients. *Int. Clin. Psychopharmacol.*, **21**(2), 87–92.

Oshima, A., Higuchi, T., Fujiwara, Y. *et al.* (1999). Questionnaire survey on the prescribing practice of Japanese psychiatrists for mood disorders. *Psychiatry Clin. Neurosci.*, **53**(suppl), S67–S72.

Philips, M. R., Lu, S. H. & Wang, R. W. (1997). Economic reforms and the acute inpatient care of patients with schizophrenia. *Am. J. Psychiatry*, **154**(9), 1228–34.

Pi, E. H., Jain, A. & Simpson, G. M. (1985). Review and survey of different prescribing practices in Asia. In C. Shagass, R. C. Josiassen, W. H. Bridger *et al.*, eds., *Biological Psychiatry*. New York, Elsevier, pp. 1536–8.

Pi, E. H., Wang, A. L. & Gray, G. E. (1993). Asian/non-Asian transcultural tricyclic antidepressant psychopharmacology: a review. *Prog. Neuropsychopharmacol. Biol. Psychiatry*, **17**(5), 691–702.

Srisurapanont, M., Garner, P., Critchley, J. & Wongpakaran, N. (2005). Benzodiazepine prescribing behaviour and attitudes: a survey among general practitioners practicing in northern Thailand. *BMC Fam. Pract.*, **6**, 27.

Udomratn, P. (1999). Prescribing habits of Thai psychiatrists in the treatment of a first episode schizophrenia. *J. Psychiatr. Assoc. Thailand*, **44**(2), 119–24.

Udomratn, P., Vasiknanonte, S., Lambert, T., Ng, C. & Freeman, N. (2004). Pattern of prescribing antipsychotic drugs in a developing country: a report from Thailand. *European Psychiatry*, **19**(suppl 1), 194S.

Wu, C. H., Chang, I. S., Tsai, F. Y. & Lin, K. M. (2007). *Using Pattern and Potential Inappropriate Use of Benzodiazepines in Taiwan*. Second International Congress of Biological Psychiatry, Santiago de Chile.

Yamawaki, S. (1999). The use and development of anxiolytics in Japan. *Eur. Neuropsychopharmacol*, **9**(suppl 6), S413–S419.

# 12

# Psychiatric inpatient psychotropic prescribing in East Asia

Chay-Hoon Tan

## Introduction

Prescribing of psychotropic drugs, such as antipsychotics, antidepressants, anxiolytics and mood stabilizers, is common in psychiatric inpatients for acute and maintenance treatment of psychiatric illness.

While no one will disagree that the psychotropic drugs should be kept to an effective minimum dosage, it is reported that Asian patients usually require a lower dosage of antipsychotic drugs than Caucasian patients (Chiu et al., 1992; Ko et al., 1989). The differences in prescribing patterns are not just observed in the dosages of psychotropic drugs, but are also seen in the types of psychotropic drugs, the use of poly-antipsychotic drugs, and the concurrent use of psychotropic drugs. Generally, prescribing patterns may be based on the following factors:

(1) biological factors including genetic susceptibility to adverse effects (Lam et al., 1995). Some researchers have argued that ethnicity may provide a marker for individual genetic variation, and that drug choice and dose should vary according to different races (Jones & Perlis, 2006);

(2) ethnicity factors (Opolka et al., 2004), in that Caucasian patients were more likely to receive an atypical antipsychotic and less likely to receive a depot injection than Latino patients (Covell et al., 2002);

(3) prescribers' professional training, where postgraduate and continuing medical education can affect the prescribing habit (Hull et al., 2005). Findings from clinical trials, particularly results from industrial sponsored clinical trials may influence prescribing patterns (Perlis et al., 2005);

(4) health care system and medical insurance (Sleath & Shih, 2003).

In 1999, the first collaborative attempt to study the prescribing of psychotropic drugs in several East Asian countries was initiated. The preliminary international

*Ethno-psychopharmacology: Advances in Current Practice*, eds. C. H. Ng, K.-M. Lin, B. S. Singh and E. Y. K. Chiu. Published by Cambridge University Press. © C. H. Ng, K.-M. Lin, B. S. Singh and E. Y. K. Chiu 2008.

collaborative research planning was started between Japan and Singapore. The collaborative group aimed to conduct "Research in East Asia on the Psychotropic Prescription Pattern," and named the acronym "REAP." The participating countries included China, Indonesia, Japan, Korea, Malaysia, Singapore, Taiwan, and Thailand. The investigators from the various countries discussed the cross-cultural issues, data collection, and study design over four consensus meetings. In 2001, the finalized standard protocol was used to gather data from all participating countries. Inpatients with the diagnosis of schizophrenia (ICD 9 or DSM IV) from seven Asian countries (China, Indonesia, Japan, Korea, Malaysia, Singapore, and Taiwan) were randomly recruited for the study from July 1 to July 30, 2001. The attending psychiatrists made clinical assessments regarding patients' psychiatric history, clinical presentation, course, treatment modality, medications, and the adverse effects of medications.

Data collection was completed and analyzed for China, Hong Kong, Taiwan, Japan, Korea, and Singapore. Comparison of the types of psychotropic medications, dosages of medications, adverse effects, and adjunct concurrent medication were done. The clinical characteristics of the patients and the use of antipsychotic drugs were also analyzed. The study enrolled a total of 2399 patients from six countries/territories of which 2368 patients were on pharmacotherapy. The mean age of all patients was 44 years although it varied in each region: the younger age group (less than 40) in China, Korea, and Taiwan; the middle age group in Singapore and Hong Kong (less than 50), to the older age group (more than 50) in Japan. The duration of illness ranged from less than a year to more than 20 years.

## Psychotropic prescribing patterns

### Antipsychotic drugs

Utilization of antipsychotic drugs varied from one region to another, depending on the availability of the drugs and the health care system (Chong *et al.*, 2004). Commonly, a higher proportion of first-generation (typical) than second-generation (atypical) antipsychotics was used across the East Asian regions. The differences in terms of types, dosages, and polypharmacy of antipsychotic drugs are described below.

### Types

Of the antipsychotic drugs prescribed, 72% were typical antipsychotics, which included haloperidol, chlorpromazine, levomepromazine, sulpiride, trifluoperazine, fluphenazine, flupentixol, and bromperidol. Use of typical drugs was associated with longer hospitalization, male gender, and clinical reports of violence or aggression. Atypical drugs only accounted for 28% of antipsychotic drugs

**Table 12.1** Percentages of prescription of atypical antipsychotic drugs in each country/territory

|                    | China | HK | Taiwan | SG | Japan | Korea |
|--------------------|-------|----|--------|----|-------|-------|
| Number of patients | 391   | 50 | 151    | 20 | 316   | 164   |
| Clozapine          | 62    | 34 | 42     | 25 | 0     | 12    |
| Olanzapine         | 3     | 48 | 7      | 10 | 11    | 18    |
| Quetiapine         | 2     | 4  | 13     | 0  | 16    | 1     |
| Zotepine           | 0     | 0  | 24     | 0  | 24    | 4     |
| Risperidone        | 33    | 14 | 15     | 65 | 45    | 66    |
| Perospirone        | 0     | 0  | 0      | 0  | 5     | 0     |

HK = Hong Kong
SG = Singapore

**Table 12.2** Percentages of daily dosages of antipsychotic drugs (mg chlorpromazine equivalent) in each country/territory

|                    | China | HK  | Taiwan | SG  | Japan | Korea | Total |
|--------------------|-------|-----|--------|-----|-------|-------|-------|
| Number of patients | 605   | 103 | 308    | 293 | 620   | 439   | 2368  |
| <300 mg            | 34    | 26  | 32     | 27  | 13    | 15    | 24    |
| 300–599 mg         | 48    | 29  | 39     | 28  | 21    | 26    | 33    |
| 600–899 mg         | 10    | 28  | 17     | 17  | 24    | 28    | 20    |
| 900–1199 mg        | 5     | 12  | 6      | 12  | 12    | 14    | 10    |
| ≥1200 mg           | 3     | 5   | 6      | 16  | 30    | 17    | 15    |

HK = Hong Kong
SG = Singapore

prescribed, which included risperidone, clozapine, zotepine, olanzapine, quetiapine, and perospirone. Use of atypical drugs was associated with positive and negative symptoms. The percentages of atypical antipsychotic use in each country/territory are shown in Table 12.1.

Across the sites, an average of 15% of inpatients received depot antipsychotic drugs (Sim *et al.*, 2004b). This was most common in Singapore (75%) followed by Taiwan (20%), Japan and China (6%). The depot antipsychotic drugs used were fluphenazine decanoate, flupenthixol decanoate, zuclopenthixol decanoate, haloperidol decanoate, pipothiazine palmitate, and fluphenazine enanthate.

### Dosages

The dosages of antipsychotic drugs differed markedly between the six sites studied (see Table 12.2). Of note, there were more than 50% of patients in China, Hong Kong, Taiwan, and Singapore taking less than 600 mg chlorpromazine-equivalents

**Table 12.3** Percentages of concurrent psychotropic drugs used in each country/territory for patients with schizophrenia

|                            | China | HK | Taiwan | SG | Japan | Korea |
|----------------------------|-------|----|--------|----|-------|-------|
| Mood stabilizers           | 25    | 32 | 37     | 31 | 36    | 26    |
| Anxiolytics and/or hypnotics | 12  | 25 | 79     | 52 | 88    | 53    |
| Antiparkinson              | 35    | 50 | 63     | 82 | 87    | 76    |
| Antidepressant             | 5     | 1  | 7      | 15 | 2     | 3     |

HK = Hong Kong
SG = Singapore

per day (CPZe). Patients in Japan, Korea, and Singapore tended to receive high-dose antipsychotic drugs (defined as more than 1000 mg of CPZe) (Sim *et al.*, 2004a). Those who received high-dose antipsychotic drugs were likely to be younger, have longer duration of admission and illness, and show violence or aggression.

## Poly-antipsychotics

Fifty-four percent of the patients received monotherapy of antipsychotic drug, whereas 46% were prescribed more than one antipsychotic drug concurrently (poly-antipsychotics). The prevalence varies from region to region. Japan has the highest rate of poly-antipsychotics (79%), followed by Singapore (72%). The results showed the use of combination high and low potency typical antipsychotic drugs, including add-on atypical to high dose typical antipsychotic drugs.

## Antidepressants

Antidepressants are used as monotherapy for depression and often during inpatient management in the six countries/territories. Anatomical Therapeutic Chemical Classification Index with Defined Daily Doses (ATC-DDD) listed 56 drugs under the category of antidepressants. The antidepressant study of the REAP survey showed that only 26 out of the 56 antidepressants were prescribed across the sites. Selective serotonic re-uptake inhibitors (SSRIs) were most frequently prescribed, followed by milnacipran, venlafaxine, amitriptyline, mirtazapine, and tryptophan. There was significant variation in the availability of antidepressants in each country, which is influenced by the registration and costs of antidepressants in each country. Among several factors, government policy for drug licensing played the decisive role in the availability of antidepressants. For example, only three newer antidepressants were available in Japan at the time of the survey. In addition to the use in depression, antidepressants were frequently used for patients with psychoses and anxiety disorders. The REAP study showed that 1–15% of patients with schizophrenia were prescribed antidepressants (see Table 12.3).

**Antianxiety and hypnotic/sedative drugs**

Benzodiazepines are efficacious and commonly used as antianxiety, hypnotic, and sedative drugs for inpatients with schizophrenia and depression. More than 50% of the inpatients with schizophrenia in the above study were prescribed with this class of drug (see Table 12.3). However, in recent years there has been growing concern about the problem of dependence and abuse. When anxiety is a symptom of another psychiatric disorder such as depression, treatment with an antidepressant is generally more effective in relieving the anxiety rather than using benzodiazepines (BZDs) as the long-term management.

**Antiparkinson drugs**

Thirty-five to eighty-seven percent of the patients studied received antiparkinson drugs. Compared to other countries, Japan and Singapore used the most of these antidotes for drug-induced extrapyramidal symptoms. This is most likely related to the frequent use of high-dosage antipsychotic drugs and poly-antipsychotics (see Table 12.3).

**Mood stabilizers**

Twenty-five to thirty-six percent of the patients studied were prescribed mood stabilizers (see Table 12.3).

## Discussion

Patients from China, Hong Kong, and Taiwan were ethnic Chinese as with the majority of patients in Singapore. This allows us to examine the prescription of psychotropic drugs in Chinese patients from the four countries/territories and compare with the patients from Japan and Korea. However, the prescribing of the type of drugs, dosages, poly-antipsychotics, concurrent psychotropics, and the use of antiparkinson drugs differ even between these four countries/territories. The prescription rate of atypical antipsychotic drugs is lowest in Singapore, which may be due to a different health care system in Singapore compared to other regions. For instance, there is no medical insurance on the use of atypical antipsychotic drugs in Singapore. On the other hand, the most frequently prescribed atypical drug in China was clozapine (see Table 12.1), which is manufactured generically in China. Another factor that may affect prescribing habits relates to clinical symptomatology. Tan *et al.* (1990) showed that drugs prescribed for long-stay inpatients were related to the patient's psychiatric symptoms and behavior. In this study of long-stay patients (N = 271), it was found that polypharmacy was higher among patients with positive symptoms, aggression, and impulsive behavior. Other factors that may affect prescribing habits include health care service systems, financing schemes, cost of drugs (see Figure 12.1), medical insurance, and cultural factors.

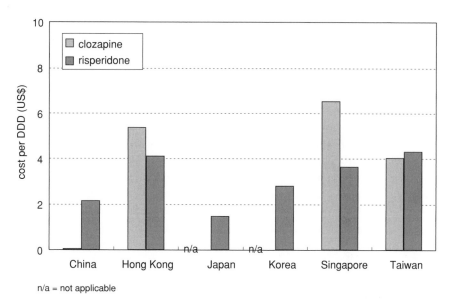

Figure 12.1    Cost of atypical antipsychotic drugs (clozapine and risperidone) in each country/territory for patients with schizophrenia

## Conclusion

The results of the REAP study raise several questions about actual prescribing practices and clinical practice guidelines used in the pharmacological treatment of schizophrenia. It is evident that the availability and cost of drugs, the health care system, and insurance policies influence the prescribing significantly. Despite the emergence of the clinical application of pharmacogenetics in psychotropic drug prescription, this study indicates the complexity of genetic versus sociocultural factors affecting prescribing patterns. Health care policy, insurance schemes, local traditions, and prescribing culture are all key issues that must all be taken into account in the management of patients with psychiatric disorders. Evidence-based medical research in the treatment of patients with schizophrenia in different ethnic groups and cultures is needed to address them.

## REFERENCES

Chiu, H., Lee, S., Leung, C. M. & Wing, Y. K. (1992). Neuroleptic prescription for Chinese schizophrenics in Hong Kong. *Aust. N. Z. J. Psychiatry*, **26**(2), 262–4.

Chong, M. Y., Tan, C. H., Fuji, S. *et al.* (2004). Antipsychotic drug prescription for schizophrenia in East Asia: a rational for change. *Psychiatry Clin. Neurosci.*, **58**, 61–7.

Covell, N. H., Jackson, C. T., Evans, A. C. & Essock, S. M. (2002). Antipsychotic prescribing practices in Connecticut's public mental health system: rates of changing medications and prescribing styles. *Schizophr. Bull.*, **28**(1), 17–29.

Hull, S. A., Aquino, P. & Cotter, S. (2005). Explaining variation in antidepressant prescribing rates in east London: a cross sectional study. *Fam. Pract.*, **22**(1), 37–42.

Jones, D. S. & Perlis, R. H. (2006). Pharmacogenetics, race, and psychiatry: prospects and challenges. *Harv. Rev. Psychiatry*, **14**(2), 92–108.

Ko, G. N., Zhang, L. D., Yan, W. W. *et al.* (1989). The Shanghai 800: prevalence of tardive dyskinesia in a Chinese psychiatric hospital. *Am. J. Psychiatry*, **146**(3), 387–9.

Lam, Y. W., Jann, M. W., Chang, W. H. *et al.* (1995). Intra- and interethnic variability in reduced haloperidol to haloperidol ratios. *J. Clin. Pharmacol.*, **35**(2), 128–36.

Opolka, J. L., Rascati, K. L., Brown, C. M. & Gibson, P. J. (2004). Ethnicity and prescription patterns for haloperidol, risperidone, and olanzapine. *Psychiatr. Serv.*, **55**(2), 151–6.

Perlis, R. H., Perlis, C. S., Wu, Y. *et al.* (2005). Industry sponsorship and financial conflict of interest in the reporting of clinical trials in psychiatry. *Am. J. Psychiatry*, **162**(10), 1957–60.

Sim, K., Su, A., Leong, J. Y. *et al.* (2004a). High dose antipsychotic use in schizophrenia: findings of the REAP (research on East Asia psychotropic prescriptions) study. *Pharmacopsychiatry*, **37**(4), 175–9.

Sim, K., Su, A., Ungvari, G. S. *et al.* (2004b). Depot antipsychotic use in schizophrenia: an East Asian perspective. *Human Psychopharmacology*, **19**, 103–9.

Sleath, B. & Shih, Y. C. (2003). Sociological influences on antidepressant prescribing. *Soc. Sci. Med.*, **56**(6), 1335–44.

Tan, C. H., Chee, K. T. & Seow, H. H. (1990). Pharmacotherapy in long-stay psychiatric patients in Singapore. *Asia Med. J.*, **33**(3), 161–7.

# 13

# Pharmaco-economic implications for Asia and other economically disadvantaged countries

Norman Sartorius

## Introduction

Several issues have to be kept in mind when reading this chapter. First, there are vast differences between the economically disadvantaged countries (Sartorius, 2001). In most of them, however, the gap between the richest and poorest parts of the population has grown over the past few decades and continues to grow. The health care for the poorest groups in the population has also become weaker and of poorer quality. In relation to pharmacotherapy this means that even when low-cost medications are made available the poor do not benefit from this, because the weakness of the health system makes it impossible for them to get to health care staff who could advise them and guide them in taking these medications.

Second, there are poor population groups in many of the rich countries, and at first glance they seem to be in a position similar to that of the poor in the Third World. This, however, is not so. The poor in the highly developed countries have access to some of the amenities that are considered exceptional and most desirable but rarely available in the Third World – such as the abundance of drinkable water and the minimal risk of contracting one of the many communicable diseases that kill people in the Third World, such as malaria. Not infrequently the poor in the industrialized countries have access to shelter and clothing provided by the often numerous humanitarian and religious organizations, such as the Salvation Army or the Emmaus organization. Emergency medical care might also be available on many occasions and there are politicians and humanists advocating their cause. The poor in the Third World rarely have any of this.

Third, the developing countries differ sharply in the speed of their development. The least developed developing countries have health budgets that do not surpass two or three dollars per inhabitant per year. In such situations access to modern

*Ethno-psychopharmacology: Advances in Current Practice*, eds. C. H. Ng, K.-M. Lin, B. S. Singh and E. Y. K. Chiu. Published by Cambridge University Press. © C. H. Ng, K.-M. Lin, B. S. Singh and E. Y. K. Chiu 2008.

technology of diagnosis and treatment becomes extremely difficult. (Sartorius & Elmsley, 2000) The rapidly developing countries on the other hand have a sizeable and growing middle-class population (and a significant number of very rich citizens) that can and does buy excellent health care in the country and abroad. This attracts many of the best government employed health workers to move to doing private practice – which also contributes to the decline of primary health care and to the increasingly difficult situation that faces the urban and rural poor in the population.

Fourth, the very competitive market makes it necessary for the pharmaceutical industry to speed up trials of medications necessary for their registration and promotion. While previously randomized control trials were conducted in a small number of sites each contributing a reasonable number of assessments, modern-day psychopharmacological research is spread widely involving numerous centers, many of them in Eastern Europe and in the developing world. Some of these centers assess effects of treatment and report on a large number of patients: yet, their data is usually included into the pool of data published in a summation report and not available for separate publication. Such trials – although financially very attractive to the staff participating in them – often exhaust the personnel resources in the centers in the Third World and thus become an additional reason for the rarity of reports about the effects of psychopharmacological medications in the developing countries.

Fifth, it is useful to remember Seige's (Snelders et al., 2006) notion of lifecycles of drugs in psychiatry and in medicine. In 1912, Seige proposed the recognition of three phases in the life of a medication: in the first, after its discovery there is much optimism and widespread use of the new compound; next follows a phase of criticism and disillusionment; finally, in a third phase, the risks and benefits of a medication are recognized and its use becomes rational. The lifecycles of drugs are, however, not synchronous in all countries. The recognition of this development is important when it comes to the development of strategies for the introduction of a medication or its removal from health services in a country. Removing a drug in the first Seige phase is very difficult and will often be accompanied by accusations of discrimination of those who do not get to use it. Introducing a drug currently in Seige phase two into a new country is also a difficult task.

## The problems

There are many obstacles that bar the way to a wide application of modern pharmacological treatment in the economically disadvantaged countries. They include the scarcity of personnel who could prescribe and supervise the application of such treatment, the omnipresent poverty, the high cost of some medications, the weakness of channels of distribution or of other arrangements that would ensure a continuing availability of medications, the stigma attached to mental illness and its numerous consequences, and finally low levels of health literacy in most developing countries. These problems are compounded by the frequency of wars and natural as well as human-made catastrophes in the Third World, by inclement climatic conditions affecting the validity of medications and by the corruption and incompetent management of the health systems in many countries.

Publications about the effects and side effects of psychopharmacological interventions in populations in the developing countries are insufficient in number and often do not meet standards of the best of evidence. Structures for an exchange of information and learning from each other, such as regular meetings and discussions, are rarely in place.

Until recently, many of the psychiatrists have received their postgraduate education abroad where they have been working with different types of patients, in a health care system that is dissimilar to the one in their own country and in a cultural setting that differs from their own. Knowledge gained abroad made it easy for them to converse with colleagues in other countries: but for work in their own country they had, upon return, to invent a practice that bore little resemblance to what they learned abroad. Many found the challenges of developing models of health care too trying: this combined with the active recruitment campaigns of governments and institutions in the developed countries with the lure of the benefits that could be theirs was so attractive that they left their country. Once settled abroad some of them offer their services as consultants to the countries from which they came, forgetting that the country of their origin might have changed since they left it and that they have left it because they could not adjust their life and practice to the conditions that prevailed in it. Sometimes they are also invited to advise nongovernmental or inter-governmental agencies about programs in their country of origin, and not infrequently they do so without consulting their colleagues who have stayed at home and valiantly tried to overcome the problems that contributed to the emigration of their consultant. Frequently the two groups (those in the country and the emigrant consultant) are covertly or overtly in conflict, criticizing one another's suggestions so that some of the excellent initiatives proposed by one of the groups never get off the ground.

The stigma attached to mental illness is pervasive and affects the lives of people with mental illness. It makes the patient reluctant to come forward and ask for help. It makes rehabilitation after an episode of illness difficult. It contributes to the loss of self-esteem of the person who has the illness, a consequence that is particularly nefarious because it often blocks full recovery. Stigma also affects the members of the family, making them reluctant to admit that one of them has a mental illness and may need treatment. It demeans institutions in which treatment is provided as well as the mental health professions, making them unattractive for the vast majority of medical graduates and nursing staff. Stigma reflects the low value that people with a mental illness have in the eyes of their community and their government. How low this value is becomes clear when governments refuse to purchase medications that serve to treat mental illness (regardless of its cost) while being prepared to pay much higher prices for medications that serve for the treatment of other illnesses. The cost of a modern antibiotic for a three-day treatment of a bacterial infection is higher than the treatment of a person with schizophrenia (using a low-cost antipsychotic drug) over two years: yet it is highly probable that the government offices would tend to buy the former, not the latter.

As a consequence of these problems, pharmacotherapy of mental disorders in the Third World, and in particular in the poorest groups of the population in economically disadvantaged countries, suffers from grave deficiencies. The knowledge about the effects and side effects of most of the (particularly modern) medications used in psychiatry is non-systematic and usually reflects the experience of practicing psychiatrists and publicity leaflets of the producers rather than a systematic evaluation of the medication in a particular sociocultural setting. Staff in general health care services know little about mental health problems and consequently neither recognize them nor become aware of their frequency and consequences. Psychiatrists are few in number and often have few opportunities to update their knowledge. Psychotropic medications are not always available and even when they are this is usually only for a relatively brief period. The population knows little about the possibilities of treatment for mental disorders and patients do not come forward very often: the usual reason for a first encounter with mental health services is an episode of serious illness with symptoms that disturb the community. Governments do not give much priority to mental health services and government officials seem to share the low opinion not only about the people with mental illness but also about psychiatry and the effectiveness of psychiatric treatment with the rest of the population. Psychotropic drugs of the newer generations are still very expensive and therefore used mainly by richer people in poor countries; when produced locally at low cost they still do not find a wide application because of the above reasons and because mental health staff are few in number and do not always feel confident about their use.

## Priorities and hopes for the future

It is difficult to say what would be the best way to improve the pharmacotherapy of mental disorders in economically disadvantaged countries. Among areas that should be examined as options for priority attention there should be at least the following.

(1) The acquisition of knowledge – using both evidence and experience – about the effectiveness and safety of psychopharmacological drugs in the setting of the country in which they are going to be used. Controlled studies, recording and exchanging information about the use of a medication, exploration of the best ways to use a medication in harmony with the sociocultural setting, collection of reports about the effects of the drug from the patients and their families, should all be seen as possible ways to acquire such knowledge.

(2) Introduction of drugs in parallel with the training of personnel who will use them. It is unlikely that all the primary health care workers will wish to deal with mental disorders: having established who among them is willing to participate in mental health care it will be necessary to make arrangements for in-service training, which will inter alia include training in the use of psychopharmacolo-gical medications. Providing training without making the medications available is not likely to be helpful; equally so, making provisions to have the medications in the hands of personnel who do not know how to use them is wasteful. In par-allel with the in-service refresher training of general and mental health service staff it is of essential importance to provide skills and knowledge needed in the provision of mental health care to students of health care professions – com-bining this instruction with a determined effort to inculcate positive attitudes to people with mental health problems and their treatment.

(3) In the development of the strategy for the improvement of pharmacotherapy, priority should be given to the introduction of medications that (a) do not have alarming or stigmatizing side effects (e.g., early and strong extrapyramidal signs; (b) have a rapid onset of action; (c) do not have to rely on laboratory examination for safe use; (d) can be applied both parenterally and perorally. The cost of medications should be carefully examined taking into account not only the effects of the drug on the symptoms of an episode of illness but also other possible savings that might accrue, for example if the treatment reduces the probability of relapses, helps to prevent suicide, and reduces the probability of family disintegration (which is more and more often the consequence of the presence of a family member with an untreated mental disorder even in traditional societies).

(4) Establishment of a neutral source of information about medications. The pro-motion of sales by the pharmaceutical industry is usually powerful and at present almost never countered by the provision of information by an organiza-tion such as the World Health Organization (WHO). The WHO has established a list of essential drugs and cooperates with centers that assemble information about side effects of medications; it has, however, until now shied away from providing, at regular intervals, well balanced reviews of treatment options and medications. Governments in some countries have tried to provide neutral

information: in most instances, however, they do so only occasionally. It could be argued that the provision of such information is expensive and requires expertise that is rarely available in the poor countries: this argument is, however, not tenable because it would be possible to establish the necessary facility for a fraction of the cost of errors that occur when such information is not available.

(5) The collaboration between mental health services and members of families of people with mental illness and their other carers is of essential importance in developing a useful and successful mental health service. Collaboration with carers is not in existence in many of the Third World countries, and in places where it exists it is at present often restricted to a one-way communication of instruction of what the carers should do to assist in the realization of the treatment plan established by the medical practitioners. Advice from carers and information about the effects of treatment can both be of great value in the treatment of individual patients and in deciding the best use of medications and other treatments in health services in general.

(6) Traditional and alternative medicine play a major role in industrialized countries, and have an even greater importance in the care of people with mental illness in the poor countries. Many of the traditional practitioners use modern psychopharmacological drugs, often in combination with traditional forms of treatment. The place of traditional medicine and the role of its practitioners is regulated differently in different countries. In some instances traditional medicine has become a regular part of the training of medical students in "Western" medical schools. In some countries the practice of traditional medicine is forbidden, in others it is given a status that is in no way different from the "Western" or "official" medicine. It is in the interests of all to establish who the traditional practitioners are, and what they do in a particular country or setting. This will allow the elaboration of arrangements that will be useful for patients and reduce the risks of the inappropriate use of medications and of delays in treatment that may otherwise occur.

## Coda

The availability of medications that are effective in the treatment of mental disorders, and safe even after extended use, is essential for the success of programs directed to the improvement of mental health care. It is essential but not sufficient because such programs must – if they are to be successful – also include efforts to improve knowledge, skills, and attitudes of health workers involved in the provision of mental health care; additional investment into mental health programs; and a resolute and continuing action against the stigma attached to mental disorders and their terrible consequences.

## REFERENCES

Sartorius, N. (2001). Psychiatry in developing countries. In F. Henn, N. Sartorius, H. Helmchen and H. Lauter, eds., *Contemporary Psychiatry*, Vol. 2. Berlin, Heidelberg, New York: Springer Verlag, pp. 247–59.

Sartorius, N. & Elmsley, R. A. (2000). Psychiatry and technological advances: implications for the developing countries. *Lancet*, **356**, 2090–2.

Snelders, S., Kaplan, C. & Peters, T. (2006). On cannabis, chloral hydrate and career cycle of psychotropic drugs in medicine, *Bull. Hist. Med.*, **80**(1), 95–114 cited in Jefferson J. W. & Greist J. H. (2006). Rethinking older psychiatric drugs. *Primary Psychiatry*, December 2006, 37–8.

# 14

# Integrating theory, practice and economics in psychopharmacology

Keh-Ming Lin, Chun-Yu Chen, Chia-Hui Chen, Jur-Shan Cheng, and Sheng-Chang Wang

Critiques and reservations regarding the role and contribution of psychotropic agents in the care of psychiatric patients notwithstanding (Moncrieff, 2001; Healy, 2002), there is little doubt that the advent of modern psychopharmacology in the 1950s has vastly and profoundly altered the landscape of psychiatry. Phenothiazines and related compounds in the past half century have enabled millions of severely mentally ill patients to escape the fate of lifelong confinement. "Antidepressants" and mood stabilizers, equally serendipitously discovered around the same time, often effectively, and at times truly miraculously, lifted millions from various forms of misery. Together they also helped to change (albeit not fast enough and still a long way to go) the public's perception of the mentally ill as well as the professions charged with their care, helping to destigmatize behavioral and emotional problems. Irrespective of the extent of their therapeutic effects, the fact that simple chemical compounds could so profoundly alter behavior was itself inspiring for a new generation of scientists, who helped to usher in a new era of intensive research for the biological substrates of psychiatric phenomena, resulting in the blossoming of biological psychiatry and neuroscience in the last few decades (Carlsson, 1988; Bloom & Kupfer, 1995).

To be sure, examined at closer range, the effect of this "paradigm shift" on the profession and for society is far more complex and nuanced. Advances on the biological front not infrequently have been regarded as threats for our field's expertise in the psychosocial domains. Concerns were often aired over the possibility of the "over-sell" of medications, offering simplistic "solutions" to problems that were almost certainly determined more by psychosocial factors than biological ones. "Medicalization" indeed is not an issue that could be easily ignored or brushed aside (Luhrmann, 2000).

*Ethno-psychopharmacology: Advances in Current Practice*, eds. C. H. Ng, K.-M. Lin, B. S. Singh and E. Y. K. Chiu. Published by Cambridge University Press. © C. H. Ng, K.-M. Lin, B. S. Singh and E. Y. K. Chiu 2008.

The reality is that, as is true in all branches of medicine, there are no magical pills nor magical cures, at least not all the time, or even most of the time. In pivotal trials that led to FDA approval of new drugs, often the response rates hovered around 50%. (Since for reasons not completely understood, placebo response rates have gone up, at times to levels similar to the active compound being tested. Thus, it has become increasingly more difficult for controlled trials to demonstrate efficacy.) Further, for those classified as responders, the "response" may not be complete. Symptom reduction may be partial, and symptomatic improvements do not necessarily translate into differences in functional status or quality of life (Jadad, 1998; Rush, Fava, Wisniewski *et al.*, 2004; Lieberman, Stroup, McEvoy *et al.*, 2005). Thus, despite the continuing and remarkable progress in psychopharmacology and in neuroscience, the majority of our patients have yet to maximally reap the fruits of the "revolution" that started half a century earlier.

That this is the case is partly reflected in the fact that there remain substantial and eminently noticeable (but often neglected) gaps between "scientific evidence" and clinical practice. Because of the gravity of such gaps, efforts have been made to promote "evidence-based medicine," practice guidelines, and treatment algorithms (Cabana, Rand, Powe *et al.*, 1999; Cook & Giacomini, 1999; McIntyre, 2002; Dawes, Davies, Gray *et al.*, 2005). However, it may be assumed that even under optimal situations, clinicians' practices will continue to deviate from best available evidence (as they should be in such a scenario). Real patients do not respond exactly as described in textbooks or research papers, which "typically" present information that describes the "typical" patients, neglecting the huge variations that invariably exist across individuals and ethnicity. This is so precisely because in studies aiming at demonstrating the efficacy of an intervention method, or at showing the validity of a hypothesis, it is indispensable that efforts be made to reduce "noise" (variance) as much as possible, whether they are industry sponsored or independently funded studies (Lebowitz & Rudorfer, 1998). Grave reservations from scholars aside, "reductionism" (i.e., focusing on one, or very few, factor(s), controlling all other factors that might influence outcome as much as possible) remains the cornerstone of scientific progress (Kendler, 2005). The challenge ahead is to reap the benefit from, but not be limited by, the insights derived from reductionistic research efforts. To this end, attempts will be made to discuss several general strategies that might be particularly crucial for reducing the gaps between research and practice, and for the further enhancement of our profession's ability to bring the fruits of our toils to the majority of our patients. These are (1) new drug discovery approaches; (2) maximizing effectiveness in practice settings; (3) clinical application of pharmacogenomics and individualized medicine; and, (4) the application of pharmaco-economics in psychopharmacology.

## New drug discovery approaches

Serendipitous discovery of the antipsychotic and antidepressant properties of chlorpromazine and imipramine led to the development of monoamine neurotransmitter theories that have guided and dominated the development of neuropsychopharmacology and subsequent drug developments (Carlsson, 1988; Bloom & Kupfer, 1995; Domino, 1999). While the paradigms have proven useful in many ways, as evidenced by the rapid proliferation of the knowledge base and the multitudes of effective therapeutic agents now available, they may also have deterred the search for alternative or innovative approaches. This notwithstanding, explorations have been initiated in a number of directions outside of the traditional monoamine neurotransmitter models (e.g., dopamine, serotonin, and norepinephrine systems). These include agents acting on glutamatergic and GABA systems (e.g., sarcosine in the treatment of schizophrenia; ketamine's effect on treatment-resistant depression), neuropeptides such as cholecystokinin (CCK), vasopressin and substance P, the hypothalamus-pituitary-adrenal axis, and the secondary messenger system (Green & Braff, 2001; Manji, Quiroz, Sporn *et al.*, 2003; Schechter, Ring, Beyer *et al.*, 2005). Although no products have yet been ready for the market or for clinical application, many of these directions are theoretically intriguing and could lead to a major breakthrough in the near future.

Another exciting new direction lies in the recent advances in psychoneuroimmunology (Leonard & Myint, 2006; Müller & Schwarz, 2006). Although neurons represent only 10% of the cells in the brain, up until recently they have received almost exclusive attention by researchers. However, recent studies have shown that the glial cells, especially the microglia, as well as endothelial cells, interact intimately with neurons (Block & Hong, 2005; Kim & de Vellis, 2005; Martinelli & Reichhart, 2005; Banks, 2006; Dantzer, 2006; Graham, Christian & Kiecolt-Glaser, 2006). They secrete a large number of substances regulating the function, development, survival, and apoptosis of neurons, including cytokines that are either pro-inflammatory or anti-inflammatory, as well as neurotrophins. Microglia cells, in particular, have been regarded as the phagocytes in the central nervous system, playing a vital role in defending the brain against assaults, yet at the same time the inappropriate or excessive activation of such defenses could also lead to deleterious effects. Based on these findings as well as clinical observations, anti-inflammatory agents such as cox-2 inhibitors and other agents that have been found to exert immuno-modulating effects, such as dextromethorphan, have been proposed for the treatment of treatment-resistant depression and schizophrenia (Rapaport, Delrahim, Bresee *et al.*, 2005; Müller & Schwarz, 2006).

The discovery of neurogenesis in certain areas (e.g., the hippocampus) of the adult brain represents a new departure from our conventional view of this organ being not regenerative past a certain age (Kempermann & Kronenberg, 2003; Ziv, Ron, Butovsky *et al.*, 2006). Although the field is still rapidly evolving, it appears that stress and depression may lead to neuronal atrophy and decreases in neurogenesis, while antidepressants and lithium show the opposite effect. Paralleling this, stress and depression have been found to depress the expression of neurotrophins that could be reversed by antidepressants (Duman & Monteggia, 2006). Emerging from these observations, the "neuronal plasticity" theory points to new ways for conceptualizing depression and for the search for new antidepressants.

Capitalizing on the phenomenal progress in new methodologies such as genomics and proteomics, major research programs also have been initiated to search for genes and pathways that might be regulated by various therapeutic agents, thereby uncovering therapeutic targets conducive to the development of new intervention methods (Hyman & Nestler, 1996; Debouck & Goodfellow, 1999). For example, by comparing microarray profiles of divergent agents with similar clinical effects, areas of convergence might emerge, which might point to the mechanism(s) crucial for treatment response (Chen & Chen, 2005b; 2005a).

In the context of all these technological advances, problems with the clinical phenotype become even more flagrant. There is little doubt that very few, if any, of our current diagnostic categories are unitary or homogeneous, creating remarkable "noise" that could easily obscure the neurobiological links that might be crucial for the understanding of the pathogenesis and treatment responses of subset(s) of patients currently being lumped together. In addition, as is true with other branches of medicine, intervention strategies might differ as diseases progress. However, such factors generally have not figured prominently in psychiatric interventions. It is clear that better ways of characterizing clinical phenotypes will need to go hand in hand with technological development before any real breakthrough could take place (Alarcón, Alegria, Bell *et al.*, 2002; Charney, Barlow, Botteron *et al.*, 2002; Lin & Lin, 2002).

## Maximizing effectiveness in practice settings

Examples abound regarding the role of serendipity in the discovery of new therapeutic approaches, which on closer examination usually turned out to be the result of clinicians paying attention to unexpected clinical effects rather than discounting them. For example, lithium was tried first for hypertension, chlorpromazine was initially developed as an anesthetic, and imipramine was originally regarded as an antihistamine and an antipsychotic agent. Without astute clinical observations, these drugs would not have found their niche, nor would clozapine have been "revived" for the benefit of millions of the most difficult to treat schizophrenic patients. Other examples include the expanded indications of newer "antidepressants" (obsessive compulsive disorder, anxiety disorders), various anti-convulsants (bipolar disorders), and atypical antipsychotics (mania, etc.).

Thus, when practice deviates from research data ("evidence-based" medicine), how do we know whether the practice needs to be modified, or if there might be a kernel of truth in the way medications are actually used? It seems that such questions arise precisely because too often we assume that once a medication is marketed, that is the end of research, whereas in fact such a point may be more appropriately regarded as the beginning of a new cycle of drug development (Stahl, 2006). Once in wide use, clinical experiences and "prescribing-based evidence" serve to provide signals for clinical "proof of concept" studies and full-scale trials, pointing to the possibility of expanding or restricting original indications. Unfortunately, too often this does not happen, and clinicians live in the limbo between "evidence-base" and the privilege of the "off label use" of medications.

For example, however defined, "polypharmacy" is rampant in all clinical settings, albeit with substantial variations across institutions and regions. Because of the bias against such "second round" of drug trials, we possess little information on the appropriateness and effectiveness (as well as danger) of various types of combination therapies (the recently completed NIMH STAR*D serves as a prominent exception). It would seem important that carefully designed studies be implemented to identify subgroups of patients who might actually benefit from such combinations.

As discussed in detail elsewhere (Lebowitz & Rudorfer, 1998; NIMH, 1998; 2005), in order to maximize the chance of demonstrating efficacy, Phase III drug trials strive for maximizing homogeneity in subject selection. Consequently, the characteristics of subjects participating in the initial clinical trials leading to the approval of a medication is typically very different from those subsequently treated in the clinical settings, in terms of outcomes, dosing strategies, and side effect profiles. In other words, the "generalizability" of efficacy type research remains to be tested, particularly when the medications are used in different population (Wells, 1999), including those with ethnic minority backgrounds (NIMH, 2001), and those residing in different countries or different parts of the world. This type of "effectiveness" research is not only important for the optimal care of the populations involved, but also represents an important source for enhancing our understanding of the way medications work (Rush *et al.*, 2004; Lieberman *et al.*, 2005), as discussed above.

## Clinical application of pharmacogenomics and individualized medicine

As discussed extensively in different chapters in this volume, the field of pharmacogenomics has come of age (Hallworth, 2004; Tucker, 2004; Weinshilboum &

Wang, 2004). At this point, we already possess extensive data on the metabolic pathways of most of the frequently prescribed medications, the enzymes involved in their transformations, methods of measuring the activity of the enzymes, characteristics of the genes encoding these enzymes, and the functional relationship of most of the genetic polymorphisms affecting enzyme activities, as well as their distributions in divergent populations. Together with recent advances in the genes encoding p-glycoprotein (MDR1) and other member transport proteins affecting first pass and penetration of drugs across the blood–brain barrier (Ishikawa, Onishi, Hirano *et al.*, 2004), we have a close to complete understanding of the genetic factors affecting the pharmacokinetic processes of many medications. On the other hand, our understanding of genes controlling putative therapeutic targets of psychotropics is less extensive. However, polymorphism in the promoter region of the serotonin transporter, termed 5-HTT gene-linked polymorphic region (5-HTTLPR), has been shown to be associated with the response of serotonin re-uptake inhibitors, as well as with behavioral traits including neuroticism, anxiety, and depression (Serretti, Benedetti, Zanardi *et al.*, 2005). Other genes including serotonin 2A receptor (Malhotra, Murphy & Kennedy, 2004), norepinephrine transporter (NET) (Yoshida, Takahashi, Higuchi *et al.*, 2004), tryptophan hydroxylase (TPH) (Serretti, Cusin, Rossini *et al.*, 2004), G-protein beta3-subunit (Gbeta3) (Lee, Cha, Ham *et al.*, 2004), and brain-derived neurotrophic factor (BDNF) (Russo-Neustadt & Chen, 2005), also have been reported.

Given that so much is already in existence, and the gravity of the problem with the current approach, which is characterized by "trial and error" and "one size fits all," it is puzzling that the much talked about "individualized medicine" has not yet been the reality. Although a number of "gene chips" have been developed (de Leon, 2006), and at least one has received FDA approval, they are rarely used outside of research settings (Roses, 2001; Kirchheiner, Bertilsson, Bruus *et al.*, 2003; Kirchheiner, Nickchen, Bauer *et al.*, 2004). The perceived complexity of the factors influencing drug response is an often cited reason for such difficulties in "translating" scientific knowledge into practice. Genotyping of multiple genes needs to be packaged together, and their interactive and/or congregate effects in determining specific drug responses need to be further examined. User-friendly computer or PDA programs will need to be developed in order for clinicians to interpret genotyping results of multiple genes that may have different meaning for different medications being considered in the clinical setting (Serretti & Smeraldi, 2004). Equipped with these tools, intervention studies could be designed to provide clinicians with "real-time" (within 24 hours) input of pharmacogenomic results, in order to factor in these test results in drug choice and dosing strategies (for example, using small starting doses of CYP2D6 substrates in CYP2D6 poor metabolizers). The clinical benefit of having pharmacogenomic input then could be compared between those treated according to such input and those being treated in the usual settings (treatment as usual). Once the "efficacy" and cost-effectiveness of the pharmacogenomic approach are demonstrated, issues related to financing, education, ethics (Ginsburg, Konstance, Allsbrook *et al.*, 2005; Landon, 2005; Perlis, Ganz, Avorn *et al.*, 2005; Paul & Fangerau, 2006), and innovation diffusion (Rogers, 1995) remain to be tackled. These "non-scientific" obstacles may prove to be even more difficult to overcome than technological challenges. However, unless they are dealt with, the population will not likely benefit from the goal of "individualized medicine."

## Application of pharmaco-economics in psychopharmacology

In an ideal world, all patients should receive the best available care, irrespective of cost. In reality, medical decisions are profoundly influenced by financial forces, both at the individual and at the societal level. However, without objective data, decision makers (patients, insurers, buyers, policy makers) may opt for "cheaper" solutions that in the long run turn out to be more expensive ("save a penny, lose a pound"). Often interventions are compared in terms of their total health cost, where the more expensive ones may be favored if it leads to less cost in other aspects of health cost (e.g., hospitalization). In psychiatry, an added challenge would be to present convincing data showing that psychiatric interventions (e.g., treatment of depression in the primary care settings) lead to less morbidity (and mortality) due to other medical afflictions, thereby achieving additional health cost savings. In addition, effective psychiatric interventions could also result in alleviation in the burden of care givers, increased productivity, decreased drain on social welfare and law enforcement workload, etc. However, such indirect benefits may be more difficult to estimate.

It should be apparent that cost–benefit estimation is intimately tied to each society's economic resources and cultural value orientations, making it even more problematic for results of such analyses to be exported from one system or region to another. For example, drugs that may be regarded as reasonably priced in the more affluent countries may be mostly out of reach in the economically disadvantaged countries. Since hospitalization is less expensive in some countries than others, savings secondary to de-institutionalization may have a differential financial impact on the system in different countries (however, such decisions should not be made primarily for cost saving, as evidenced by the disaster in the American system). For these reasons, it is crucial that research in the areas of pharmaco-economics and health economics be regarded as of high priority not only in the developed countries, but even more so in the less developed countries, and sociocultural factors carefully considered in such efforts (Kremer, 2002; Matowe & Katerere, 2002; Aaserud, Dahlgren, Kösters *et al.*, 2006).

## Conclusion

Despite amazing progress in psychopharmacology in the last half century, a substantial proportion of our patients fail to respond to our treatment, or do not maximally benefit from these modern advances. There are also profound gaps between research based "evidence" and clinical practices, which are further complicated and broadened in cross-cultural settings (which mean the majority of the world's populations). To bridge these gaps, and to ensure that patients benefit from modern advances in psychopharmacology and neuroscience, we need to not only search for innovative approaches to speed up drug discovery efforts; critically examine patterns of clinical responses, especially where they deviate from textbooks or "evidence-base," to better understand how responses might vary in different clinical settings (effectiveness research) and to search for new inspirations; and to capitalize on progress in clinical pharmacogenomics to realize the goals of individualized medicine. Finally, pharmaco-economics should also feature prominently in searching for optimal intervention methods for individuals as well as for communities. Ethnicity and culture (as well as social factors) represent important considerations in all these directions.

### REFERENCES

Aaserud, M., Dahlgren, A. T., Kösters, J. P. *et al.* (2006). Pharmaceutical policies: effects of reference pricing, other pricing, and purchasing policies. *Cochrane Database Syst. Rev.*, **19**(2), CD005979.

Alarcón, R. D., Alegria, M., Bell, C. C. *et al.* (2002). Chapter 6. Beyond the funhouse mirrors. In D. J. Kupfer, M. B. First and D. A. Regier, eds., *A Research Agenda for DSM-V.* American Psychiatric Association, 219–81.

Banks, W. A. (2006). The blood–brain barrier in psychoneuroimmunology. *Neurol. Clin.*, **24**(3), 413–19.

Block, M. L. & Hong, J. S. (2005). Microglia and inflammation-mediated neurodegeneration: multiple triggers with a common mechanism. *Prog. Neurobiol.*, **76**(2), 77–98.

Bloom, F. E. & Kupfer, D. J., eds. (1995). *Psychopharmacology: the Fourth Generation of Progress.* New York: Raven Press.

Cabana, M. D., Rand, C. S., Powe, N. R. *et al.* (1999). Why don't physicians follow clinical practice guidelines? A framework for improvement. *J.A.M.A.*, **282**(15), 1458–65.

Carlsson, A. (1988). The current status of the dopamine hypothesis of schizophrenia. *Neuropsychopharmacology*, **1**(3), 179–86.

Charney, D. S., Barlow, D. H., Botteron, K. *et al.* (2002). Chapter 2. Neuroscience research agenda to guide development of a pathophysiologically based classification system. In D. J. Kupfer, M. B. First and D. A. Regier, eds., *A Research Agenda for DSM-V.* American Psychiatric Association, pp. 31–84.

Chen, M.-L. & Chen, C.-H. (2005a). Comparative proteome analysis revealed up-regulation of transthyretin in rat brain under chronic clozapine treatment. *J. Psychiatric Res.*, **41**(1/2), 63–8.

Chen, M.-L. & Chen, C.-H. (2005b). Microarray analysis of differentially expressed genes in rat frontal cortex under chronic risperidone treatment. *Neuropsychopharmacology*, **30**(2), 268–77.

Cook, D. & Giacomini, M. (1999). The trials and tribulations of clinical practice guidelines. *J.A.M.A.*, **281**(20), 1950–1.

Dantzer, R. (2006). Cytokine, sickness behavior, and depression. *Neurol. Clin.*, **24**(3), 441–60.

Dawes, M., Davies, P., Gray, A. *et al.* (2005). *Evidence-Based Practice: A Primer for Health Care Professionals*. Edinburgh: Elsevier Churchill Livingstone.

de Leon, J. (2006). AmpliChip CYP450 test: personalized medicine has arrived in psychiatry. *Expert Rev. Mol. Diagn.*, **6**, 277–86.

Debouck, C. & Goodfellow, P. N. (1999). DNA microarrays in drug discovery and development. *Nat. Genet.*, **21**, 48–50.

Domino, E. F. (1999). History of modern psychopharmacology: a personal view with an emphasis on antidepressants. *Psychosom. Med.*, **61**(5), 591–8.

Duman, R. S. & Monteggia, L. M. (2006). A neurotrophic model for stress-related mood disorders. *Biol. Psychiatry*, **59**(12), 1116–27.

Ginsburg, G. S., Konstance, R. P., Allsbrook, J. S. & Schulman, K. A. (2005). Implications of pharmacogenomics for drug development and clinical practice. *Arch. Intern. Med.*, **165**(20), 2331–6.

Graham, J., Christian, L. & Kiecolt-Glaser, J. (2006). Stress, age, and immune function: toward a lifespan approach. *J. Behav. Med.*, **29**, 389–400.

Green, M. F. & Braff, D. L. (2001). Translating the basic and clinical cognitive neuroscience of schizophrenia to drug development and clinical trials of antipsychotic medications. *Biol. Psychiatry* **49**(4), 374–84.

Hallworth, M. J. (2004). The drugs dont work: pharmacogenomics – clinical biochemistry's future? *Ann. Clin. Biochem.*, **41**, 260–2.

Healy, D. (2002). *The Creation of Psychopharmacology*. Cambridge, MA: Harvard University Press.

Hyman, S. E. & Nestler, E. J. (1996). Initiation and adaptation: a paradigm for understanding psychotropic drug action. *Am. J. Psychiatry*, **153**(2), 151–62.

Ishikawa, T., Onishi, Y., Hirano, H. *et al.* (2004). Pharmacogenomics of drug transporters: a new approach to functional analysis of the genetic polymorphisms of ABCB1 (P-glycoprotein/MDR1). *Biol. Pharm. Bull.*, **27**, 939–48.

Jadad, A. R. (1998). *Randomised Controlled Trials: A User's Guide*. London: BMJ Publishing Group.

Kempermann, G. & Kronenberg, G. (2003). Depressed new neurons? Adult hippocampal neurogenesis and a cellular plasticity hypothesis of major depression. *Biol. Psychiatry*, **54**(5), 499–503.

Kendler, K. S. (2005). Toward a philosophical structure for psychiatry. *Am. J. Psychiatry*, **162**(3), 433–40.

Kim, S. U. & de Vellis, J. (2005). Microglia in health and disease. *J. Neurosci. Res.*, **81**(3), 302–13.

Kirchheiner, J., Bertilsson, L., Bruus, H. *et al.* (2003). Individualized medicine – implementation of pharmacogenetic diagnostics in antidepressant drug treatment of major depressive disorders. *Pharmacopsychiatry*, **36**, 235–43.

Kirchheiner, J., Nickchen, K., Bauer, M. *et al.* (2004). Pharmacogenetics of antidepressants and antipsychotics: the contribution of allelic variations to the phenotype of drug response. *Mol. Psychiatry*, **9**, 442–73.

Kremer, M. (2002). Pharmaceuticals and the developing world. *J. Econ. Perspect.*, **16**(4), 67–90.

Landon, M. R. (2005). Ethics and policy perspectives on personalized medicine in the post-genomic era. *J. Biolaw Bus.*, **8**(3), 28–36.

Lebowitz, B. D. & Rudorfer, M. V. (1998). Treatment research at the millennium: from efficacy to effectiveness. *J. Clin. Psychopharmacol.*, **18**(1), 1.

Lee, H.-J., Cha, J.-H., Ham, B.-J. *et al.* (2004). Association between a G-protein bold beta3 subunit gene polymorphism and the symptomatology and treatment responses of major depressive disorders. *Pharmacogenomics J.*, **4**, 29–33.

Leonard, B. E. & Myint, A. (2006). Changes in the immune system in depression and dementia: causal or coincidental effects? *Dialogues Clin. Neurosc.*, **8**(2), 163–74.

Lieberman, J. A., Stroup, T. S., McEvoy, J. P. *et al.* (2005). Effectiveness of antipsychotic drugs in patients with chronic schizophrenia. *N. Engl. J. Med.*, **353**(12), 1209–23.

Lin, K.-M. & Lin, M. (2002). Chapter 5. Challenging the Myth of a Culture-free Nosological System. In K. Kurasaki, S. Okazaki and S. Sue, eds., *Asian American Mental Health: Assessment Theories and Methods*. New York: Plenum, pp. 67–73.

Luhrmann, T. M. (2000). *Of Two Minds: The Growing Disorder in American Psychiatry*. New York: Knopf.

Malhotra, A. K., Murphy, G. M., Jr. & Kennedy, J. L. (2004). Pharmacogenetics of psychotropic drug response. *Am. J. Psychiatry*, **161**(5), 780–96.

Manji, H. K., Quiroz, J. A., Sporn, J. *et al.* (2003). Enhancing neuronal plasticity and cellular resilience to develop novel, improved therapeutics for difficult-to-treat depression. *Biol. Psychiatry*, **53**(8), 707–42.

Martinelli, C. & Reichhart, J.-M. (2005). Evolution and integration of innate immune systems from fruit flies to man: lessons and questions. *J. Endotoxin Res.*, **11**, 243–8.

Matowe, L. & Katerere, D. R. (2002). Globalization and pharmacy: a view from the developing world. *Ann. Pharmacother.*, **36**(5), 936–8.

McIntyre, J. S. (2002). Usefulness and limitations of treatment guidelines in psychiatry. *World Psychiatry*, **1**(3), 186–9.

Moncrieff, J. (2001). Are antidepressants overrated? A review of methodological problems in antidepressant trials. *J. Nerv. Ment. Dis.*, **189**(5), 288–95.

Müller, N. & Schwarz, M. J. (2006). Neuroimmune endocrine crosstalk in schizophrenia and mood disorders. *Expert Rev. Neurother.*, **6**, 1017–38.

NIMH (1998). *Bridging Science and Service*. A report by the National Advisory Mental Health Council's Clinical Treatment and Services Research Workgroup. Washington, D.C.

NIMH (2001). *An Investment in America's Future: Racial/Ethnic Diversity in Mental Health Research Careers*. Report of the National Advisory Mental Health Council Workgroup on

Racial/Ethnic Diversity in Research Training and Health Disparities Research. Washington, D.C.

NIMH (2005). *Treatment Research in Mental Illness: Improving the Nation's Public Mental Health Care through NIMH Funded Interventions Research.* Report of the National Advisory Mental Health Council's Workgroup on Clinical Trials. Washington, D.C.

Paul, N. W. & Fangerau, H. (2006). Why should we bother? Ethical and social issues in individualized medicine. *Curr. Drug Targets*, **7**, 1721–7.

Perlis, R. H., Ganz, D. A., Avorn, J. *et al.* (2005). Pharmacogenetic testing in the clinical management of schizophrenia: a decision-analytic model. *J. Clin. Psychopharmacol.*, **25**(5), 427–34.

Rapaport, M. H., Delrahim, K. K., Bresee, C. J. *et al.* (2005). Celecoxib augmentation of continuously ill patients with schizophrenia. *Biol. Psychiatry*, **57**(12), 1594–6.

Rogers, E. M. (1995). *Diffusion of Innovations.* New York: Free Press.

Roses, A. D. (2001). Pharmacogenetics. *Hum. Mol. Genet.*, **10**, 2261–7.

Rush, A. J., Fava, M., Wisniewski, S. R. *et al.* (2004). Sequenced treatment alternatives to relieve depression (STAR*D): rationale and design. *Controlled Clinical Trials*, **25**(1), 119–42.

Russo-Neustadt, A. A. & Chen, M. J. (2005). Brain-derived neurotrophic factor and antidepressant activity. *Curr. Pharm. Des.*, **11**, 1495–510.

Schechter, L. E., Ring, R. H., Beyer, C. E. *et al.* (2005). Innovative approaches for the development of antidepressant drugs: current and future strategies. *NeuroRx*, **2**(4), 590–611.

Serretti, A. & Smeraldi, E. (2004). Neural network analysis in pharmacogenetics of mood disorders. *BMC Med. Genet.*, **5**(1), 27.

Serretti, A., Cusin, C., Rossini, D. *et al.* (2004). Further evidence of a combined effect of SERTPR and TPH on SSRIs response in mood disorders. *Am. J. Med. Genet. B Neuropsychiatr. Genet.*, **129B**(1), 36–40.

Serretti, A., Benedetti, F., Zanardi, R. & Smeraldi, E. (2005). The influence of serotonin transporter promoter polymorphism (SERTPR) and other polymorphisms of the serotonin pathway on the efficacy of antidepressant treatments. *Prog. Neuro psychopharmacol. Biol. Psychiatry*, **29**(6), 1074–84.

Stahl, S. M. (2006). Finding what you are not looking for: strategies for developing novel treatments in psychiatry. *NeuroRx*, **3**(1), 3–9.

Tucker, G. (2004). Pharmacogenetics – expectations and reality. *B.M.J.* **329**(7456), 4–6.

Weinshilboum, R. & Wang, L. (2004). Pharmacogenomics: bench to bedside. *Nat Rev. Drug Discov.*, **3**(9), 739–48.

Wells, K. B. (1999). Treatment research at the crossroads: the scientific interface of clinical trials and effectiveness research. *Am. J. Psychiatry*, **156**(1), 5–10.

Yoshida, K., Takahashi, H., Higuchi, H. *et al.* (2004). Prediction of antidepressant response to milnacipran by norepinephrine transporter gene polymorphisms. *Am. J. Psychiatry*, **161**(9), 1575–80.

Ziv, Y., Ron, N., Butovsky, O. *et al.* (2006). Immune cells contribute to the maintenance of neurogenesis and spatial learning abilities in adulthood. *Nat. Neurosci.*, **9**(2), 268–75.

# 15

# Research directions in ethno-psychopharmacology

Chee H. Ng

Inter-individual and inter-ethnic differences in drug response have been regularly found in clinical practice. This is not surprising given the remarkable diversity in genetic polymorphisms, environmental factors, cultural contexts, and treatment settings. Although some of the key research reports and pertinent data have been summarized in previous chapters, systematically conducted studies in this field remain scarce, sporadic, and lacking in consistency (Lin *et al.*, 1999). Ethnic and sociocultural variables are rarely analyzed or controlled in published studies on drug effects. Such paucity of cross-ethnic data exists even though there is widespread use of psychotropics to treat people with mental disorders globally. There are compelling reasons why research in this area is very much needed to understand cross-cultural differences in psychopharmacology better. There is significant demographic shift with increasing multicultural populations in both Western and non-Western societies. As a consequence, there has been a significant growth of cultural psychiatry internationally. For instance, Asians represent more than half of the global population, and all the major psychotropics are widely prescribed in Asia. With increasing pressure on the health dollar, there is a need to improve the cost-effectiveness of pharmacotherapeutic agents by reducing the morbidity and mortality of medication side effects occurring in drug-sensitive individuals and populations (e.g., in many parts of Asia). Given that factors involved in determining inter-ethnic differences in drug response are often similar to those responsible for inter-individual variations, advances in cross-ethnic psychopharmacology can contribute to greater understanding of individual differences as well (Lin *et al.*, 1993).

Despite the plethora of new drug developments in neuroscience, most clinical drug trials are conducted in predominantly Caucasian populations even though they are used frequently in non-Caucasian populations. There is an urgent need to clarify the appropriateness of extrapolating research data of clinical drug trials

*Ethno-psychopharmacology: Advances in Current Practice*, eds. C. H. Ng, K.-M. Lin, B. S. Singh and E. Y. K. Chiu. Published by Cambridge University Press. © C. H. Ng, K.-M. Lin, B. S. Singh and E. Y. K. Chiu 2008.

derived from one population to another. As ethnicity is emerging to be an equally important variable, like age, gender, physical status (renal and hepatic impairment), and pregnancy, it should be considered in psychopharmacotherapy and be incorporated into new drug development programs. Increasingly, national drug regulatory bodies are considering population-specific data before approving the use of new drugs in their countries (Lesko & Woodcock, 2002). Data on drug dosages, efficacy, and toxicity in different ethnic groups are needed because the global population will ultimately be exposed to these drugs. Furthermore, polypharmacy of both prescribed and non-prescribed drugs is commonplace especially in non-Western cultures, leading to high potential of drug–drug, or drug–herb, or drug–substance interactions. Such factors are seldom studied systematically.

## Ethno-psychopharmacology in the new era of pharmacogenetics

The therapeutic and adverse effects of psychotropic drugs are largely determined by genetic factors as described in Chapter 5. Recent advances in pharmacogenetics and genotyping technology have highlighted the potential utility in predicting metabolic phenotypes, risks for side effects, and likelihood of drug response for the individual patient. Employing genotyping to guide individual choice and dosing of psychotropic medications is becoming a promising direction in psychopharmacology to optimize clinical response and to prevent excessive side effects. The systematic characterization of the nature and function of pharmacokinetic and pharmacodynamic genotypes to determine the best drug at the right dose and administer to the right patient could become a reality sooner rather than later. There is, however, still much to be learned before genotyping becomes a standard means of deciding the right prescription in routine clinical practice. To what extent the advances in pharmacogenetics can produce more precise and rational prescribing in clinical practice requires more research.

Challenges in pharmacogenetic research are numerous, not in the least the diversity and heterogeneity of genotypes within subpopulations and ethnic differences in the rate of individual polymorphisms. Each genotype may only contribute to a small proportion of the overall variance in treatment response and adverse effects. Studies need to be adequately powered that take into account the uneven distribution of genetic variants in comparative treatment groups (Ng et al., 2004). Therapeutic response to a psychotropic drug may also be determined by multiple genes including those controlling drug metabolism, drug transporter systems, and drug receptors, which in turn may have genetic subvariants affecting clinical response. DNA microarray technology is currently available that is capable of determining genotypes in hundreds of polymorphic loci for multiple subjects. However, data

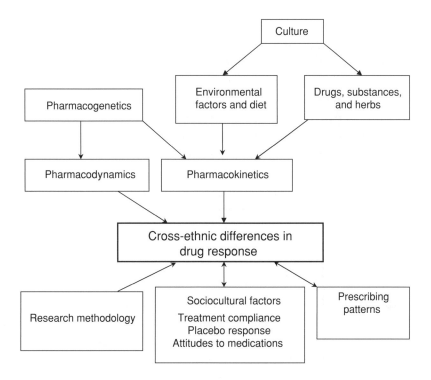

Figure 15.1 Cross-ethnic variations in psychopharmacology: influences of genetics, environment, and culture

analysis methodology for testing the reliability of genotype and clinical interaction has not been systematically developed.

Prediction of drug response using genotyping in the complex clinical environment needs to consider the broader context together with other metabolic, clinical, cultural, and environmental variables that impinge on drug response. The expressions of polymorphic genes that control brain function and drug-metabolizing enzymes interacting with environmental factors remain poorly understood. In addition, cross-cultural attributes, attitudes to medication, drug adherence, dietary factors, and the use of herbal and other traditional treatment may impact upon drug response and can be important and consequential in psychopharmacotherapy. Psychotropic treatment response can be affected further by local clinical guidelines and prescribing practices. As outlined in Chapters 11 and 12, prescribing patterns that vary cross-nationally are likely to be determined by sociocultural, economic, and systemic factors rather than any intrinsic biological function in different populations.

As shown in Figure 15.1, variations in the ethnic response to drugs are related to many interlinking factors. Genetic factors that control both pharmacokinetics and pharmacodynamics of psychotropic drugs are subject to marked variation between individuals and between ethnic groups. These genetic polymorphisms control both the function of drug-metabolizing enzymes as well as drug targets including transporters, receptors, and intracellular mechanisms. The expression of these genes is significantly modified by a range of environmental factors, including dietary factors, herbal medication, concomitant medication, and other substances (Lin & Smith, 2000). On the other hand, the importance of cultural factors, which are frequently underestimated and neglected, may also lead to differential response to psychopharmacotherapeutics. Patient attitudes to drugs, expectation of response, placebo effect, medication compliance, the doctor–patient relationship factors, illness behavior, and other psychological and social factors impinge on both the therapeutic and adverse effects experienced by patients (Ng *et al.*, 2004). Furthermore, prescribing biases of the clinician may often determine the type and the dosage of the medication during treatment initiation and maintenance, which may lead to differences in response. Methodological factors have also been identified to be a source of variation and inconsistency in research data for ethno-psychopharmacology (Pi, 1998). In a sense, practically all factors affecting pharmacological responses can be either directly or indirectly influenced by cultural or ethnic factors.

## Aiming for an integrated model of ethno-psychopharmacology

The field of ethno-psychopharmacology examines the biological and non-biological variability across ethnicity, culture, and environment in pharmacological treatments in psychiatry. The presence of inter-individual, inter-ethnic, and cross-cultural variation in psychotropic response highlights the richness in both biological and cultural processes affecting clinical psychopharmacotherapy. Treatment outcomes are influenced by genetic and non-genetic factors, and observed differences found between groups may be correlates of either biological or environmental factors, or both. To understand the complexity of cross-cultural determinants in psychopharmacology requires the consideration of multiple variables including genetic, metabolic, environmental/dietary, sociocultural, and systemic factors that play a role in therapeutic response.

It is important to emphasize in this regard that such diversity in both biological and psychosocial variables is found not only between ethnic and cultural groups but also between individuals within an ethnic subgroup. Of note, frequency differences in genetic polymorphisms although apparent across populations, may not apply to the individual patient because of intra-group variation. Due to both inter-ethnic and inter-individual differences, stereotypic clinical and research interpretations narrowly based on ethnic or racial categories should be avoided (Lin & Smith, 2000). Ethnicity per se cannot accurately specify individual metabolism or the need for specific dosing. However, there is the need to emphasize biological diversity and to question whether standard dosing is appropriate for each individual. It stands to reason that ethnicity remains a useful and important clinical pointer in pharmacotherapy to predict the probability of high or low metabolic capacity. In this sense, it could be regarded like other clinical variables such as age, gender, hepatic/renal function, weight, and physical status in tailoring an individual treatment regime.

Therefore, ethno-cultural differences point to the wide variability of biopsychosocial factors affecting psychopharmacological response not only between groups but also between individuals. Furthermore, the expressions of these genetic/biological and sociocultural entities are not static, nor are the interrelationships between them linear, as they are constantly being modified by the wider environmental context. Change in one factor can alter other relevant variables in ways that may change the qualitative and quantitative clinical outcomes.

The dynamic and interactive nature of these factors is not confined to one level or system. For instance, an Asian subject whose genotype consists of low functioning alleles for drug-metabolizing enzymes, expresses poor metabolizer (PM) phenotype and experiences severe drug side effects due to impaired drug metabolism. The subject develops markedly negative attitudes towards "Western" medications (when the culturally based fears that such medicines are too strong turns out to be true), becomes non-compliant, and drops out of treatment leading to a poor clinical outcome. Another example is the frequent use of traditional herbal medications by a Chinese patient (a culturally consistent practice) subsequently converts the patient from an extensive metabolizer (EM) to a PM because the herbs inhibit the cytochrome enzymes. Due to unexpected side effects from increased serum levels of a medication being prescribed, the treating doctor misperceives that Chinese patients are drug sensitive, and develops a bias towards prescribing low dosages (sub-therapeutic doses) for all patients of similar ethnic background. Furthermore, cultural variations may exist in the biopsychosocial determinants of psychiatric disorders resulting in differential illness expression. Hence, the clinical response of psychotropic agents both in terms of therapeutic and adverse effects is likely to be experienced differently. It is thus evident that environmental and cultural variables can exert their effects at the biological level. Vice versa, genetic/biological factors may also alter cultural practice and behavior, which can influence drug response.

Therefore it can be argued that there is an interactional relationship between these dynamic variables occurring from micro (molecular) to macro (sociocultural) levels. The complexity in conceptualizing the impact of multilevel diversity on pharmacotherapy can be brought together in an integrated model as a basis for systematic description and research. Applying a systematic and integrated approach,

**Table 15.1** Development of an international collaborative ethno-psychopharmacology research program

- Establish links with key collaborators in the region
- Using standardized methodology across all study sites
- Identify valid and reliable research instruments
- Develop training packages for all regional investigators
- Implement the research projects in respective sites
- Arrange for common laboratory for analyses or apply cross-laboratory checks
- Controlling for appropriate variables e.g., concomitant medications, diet

perhaps most effectively through an international collaborative research program, can significantly contribute to the scientific advancement of this field. Such an approach is outlined in Table 15.1. Previous examples of such collaboration have included recent studies in antipsychotics and antidepressants between Caucasian and Chinese ethnicities across different countries (Ng *et al.*, 2005; Ng *et al.*, 2006a; Ng *et al.*, 2006b). Potentially more studies in the future can map out the control parameters and the relative importance of each determinant in modifying the clinical response to psychotropic drugs.

## Future research directions

The aims of future research programs to advance the emerging field of international psychopharmacology should be directed to several overarching goals in addition to answering specific research questions. The first key objective is to apply a systematic method in studying the integrated model of cross-cultural psychopharmacology to increase the understanding of the multilevel processes involved in pharmacotherapeutic response. The second key objective is to establish the evidence base that psychopharmacotherapy needs to be adapted to match both the biological and socio-cultural diversity of individual patients. In addition, to enable flexible individual tailoring of psychotropic drug therapy, further necessary prerequisites include optimal drug "delivery" based on best clinical prescribing practice, favorable patient acceptance, and adequate drug availability.

The specific research questions that have important clinical implications include the following:

- What are the variations in pharmacokinetics and pharmacodynamics of new generation psychotropics in different ethnic and cultural groups? Are clinical drug trial data from specific population subgroups required before new drug approval is given?

- Are dose adjustments for new antidepressants and antipsychotics necessary across ethnic groups?
- What are the expected differences in side-effect profiles between ethnic groups, in particular with selective serotonic re-uptake inhibitors and atypical antipsychotics? Can the morbidity of medication side effects be reduced, hence increasing treatment compliance and effectiveness?
- What is the impact of genetic variation in driving such differences in drug response between ethnic groups? Is there a role for genotyping in predicting clinical drug response in psychiatry and preventing severe drug reactions?
- Do culturally based attitudes have a significant influence on both therapeutic and adverse effects of psychotropics? Can these attitudes be reliably quantified cross-culturally?
- What are the similarities and differences in prescribing patterns across different countries that may be determined by local and systemic service factors? How can pharmacotherapy clinical guidelines and policy facilitate best practice to treat biologically and culturally diverse individuals?
- To what extent do environmental variables such as diet and substances have an influence in pharmacotherapy? Can we minimize the adverse impact of drug–substance and drug–herb interactions?

## Conclusions

In summary, by examining the relevant aspects of ethno-psychopharmacology and conducting new research derived from cross-cultural research projects, greater progress in the knowledge and practice in this field can be made. The advances in pharmacogenetics have provided a useful tool in predicting metabolic phenotypes, risks for side effects and likelihood of drug response for the individual patient. Employing genotyping to guide individual choice and dosing of psychotropic medications is a promising direction in psychopharmacology in the future to enable optimal clinical response and to prevent excessive side effects. However, the potential use of pharmacogenetics needs to take into consideration the significant cultural and environmental factors that also impinge on response to medications within the broader systemic variables. This is an important consideration for further scientific research, clinical guideline development, and educational programs to ensure evidence-based clinical practice is grounded on adequate understanding of biological and sociocultural influence on psychopharmacology. Having a greater understanding of the role and impact of genetic/biological, environment, and cultural factors on psychopharmacotherapeutic response, may hopefully improve the treatment outcomes for different individuals and diverse ethnic groups.

## REFERENCES

Lesko, L. & Woodcock, J. (2002). Pharmacogenetic-guided drug development: regulatory perspective. *Pharmacogenomics J.*, **2**, 20–4.

Lin, K. M. & Smith, M. W. (2000). Psychopharmacotherapy in the context of culture and ethnicity. In P Ruiz ed., *Ethnicity and Psychopharmacology*. Washington, DC: American Psychiatric Press, pp. 1–36.

Lin, K. M., Poland, R. E. & Silver, B. (1993). Overview: the interface between psychobiology and ethnicity. In K. M. Lin, R. E. Poland & G Nakasaki, eds., *Psychopharmacology and Psychobiology of Ethnicity*. Washington DC: American Psychiatric Press, pp. 11–35.

Lin, K. M., Smith, M. W. & Mendoza, R. P. (1999). Psychopharmacology in cross-cultural psychiatry. In J. M. Herrera, W. B. Lawson & J. J. Sramek, eds., *Cross-Cultural Psychiatry*. New York: Wiley, pp. 45–52.

Ng, C. H., Schweitzer, I., Norman, T. & Easteal, S. (2004). The emerging role of pharmacogenetics: implications for clinical psychiatry. *Aust. N. Z. J. Psychiatry*, **38**, 483–9.

Ng, C. H., Chong, S. A., Lambert, T. *et al.* (2005). An interethnic comparison study of clozapine dosage, clinical response and plasma levels. *Int. Clin. Psychopharmacol.*, **20**, 163–8.

Ng, C. H., Norman, T. R., Naing, K. O. *et al.* (2006a). A comparison study of sertraline dosages and response in Chinese versus Caucasian patients. *J. Int. Clin. Psychopharmacol.*, **21**, 87–92.

Ng, C. H., Easteal, S., Tan, S. *et al.* (2006b). Serotonin transporter polymorphisms and clinical response to sertraline across ethnicities. *Prog. Neuropsychopharmacol. Biol. Psychiatry*, **30**, 953–7.

Pi, E. H. (1998). Transcultural psychopharmacology: present and future. *Psychiatry Clin. Neurosci.*, **52**, S185–S187.

# Index